BORDERLINE PERSONALITY DISORDER

A JOHNS HOPKINS PRESS HEALTH BOOK

BORDERLINE PERSONALITY DISORDER

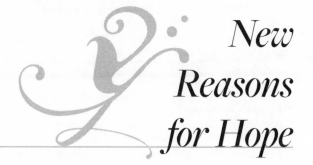

New Reasons for Hope

Francis Mark
MONDIMORE, M.D.

Patrick
KELLY, M.D.

The Johns Hopkins University Press
Baltimore

6/7/12
Lan
$ 19.95

© 2011 The Johns Hopkins University Press
All rights reserved. Published 2011
Printed in the United States of America on acid-free paper
9 8 7 6 5 4 3 2 1

The Johns Hopkins University Press
2715 North Charles Street
Baltimore, Maryland 21218-4363
www.press.jhu.edu

LIBRARY OF CONGRESS CATALOGING-IN-PUBLICATION DATA
Mondimore, Francis Mark, 1953–
    Borderline personality disorder : new reasons for hope /
Francis Mark Mondimore and Patrick Kelly.
        p. cm. (a Johns Hopkins Press health book)
    Includes bibliographical references and index.
    ISBN-13: 978-1-4214-0313-7 (hardcover : alk. paper)
    ISBN-10: 1-4214-0313-7 (hardcover : alk. paper)
    ISBN-13: 978-1-4214-0314-4 (pbk. : alk. paper)
    ISBN-10: 1-4214-0314-5 (pbk. : alk. paper)
    1. Borderline personality disorder — Popular works.   I. Kelly, Patrick, 1978–
II. Title.
    RC569.5.B67M66 2011
    616.85'852—dc22   2011008903

A catalog record for this book is available from the British Library.

Figures 4.2 and 10.1 are by Jacqueline Schaffer.

Special discounts are available for bulk purchases of this book. For more information, please contact Special Sales at 410-516-6936 or specialsales@press.jhu.edu.

The Johns Hopkins University Press uses environmentally friendly book materials, including recycled text paper that is composed of at least 30 percent post-consumer waste, whenever possible.

CONTENTS

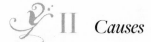

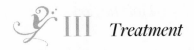

III   *Treatment*

IV   *How to Cope, How to Help*

ACKNOWLEDGMENTS

The authors would like to acknowledge many individuals who contributed to this project with their support and wisdom. First and foremost, thanks to Lynn Stanton, MSW, LCSW, of the Carolinas Healthcare System, whose clinical expertise in the treatment of borderline personality disorder patients was of invaluable help to us in writing every page of this book. Thanks as well to Daniel Buccino, LCSW, Kathleen Evans, MSN, APRN, PMH/BC, and Alice Weisko, Psy.D., and our other colleagues at the Community Psychiatry Program of the Johns Hopkins Bayview Medical Center for their expert feedback on the psychotherapy sections of the book; a more passionate and compassionate group of psychotherapists surely cannot be found anywhere. Thanks to Sina Saidi, M.D., and Chester Schmidt, M.D., for their encouragement during early phases of the project. Any errors are our own.

Thanks to medical illustrator Jacqueline Schaffer for her elegant drawings and to Nelson Donegal, Ph.D., for permission to adapt and use the fMRI image from his important neuroimaging work.

Many thanks to Jacqueline Wehmueller, executive editor for the Johns Hopkins University Press, who first suggested this book; without her patient persuasion and gentle prodding to take on the subject and persevere in its writing, the book simply wouldn't have happened.

F. M.: I would like to thank Joe Craig and Larry Tilson, who graciously allowed me to turn their Blue Ridge Mountain cabin into a writers' retreat last summer, and of course, my husband, Jay Rubin, for making sure that I don't take myself too seriously.

P. K.: I would like to thank my family for encouraging me to add what has turned into a wonderful literary journey to an already overfilled schedule. Most of all I would like to thank my husband, Michael Lindsay, for his unwavering patience, support, and encouragement throughout this process.

INTRODUCTION

Individuals who receive a diagnosis of borderline personality disorder have many problems in their emotional lives, in their relationships, and in their behaviors. These problems interact with, exacerbate, and sustain one another. This complexity makes it difficult to know where to start in understanding these individuals better, or how to help them and those who care about them. In this book, we will tease apart this complexity a little at a time to help you grasp these problems better and learn how to be helpful.

If *you* have been diagnosed with borderline personality disorder, or BPD, we hope that in reading this book, you will understand yourself better, learn how to help your treatment team help you, and begin building healthier relationships and a happier life.

If someone you care about has received a diagnosis of BPD, this book can guide you in understanding the experiences of that person well enough to know how to help and, just as importantly, to learn which problems you will *not* be able to help with. We also talk about how a person who has BPD gets into treatment.

We believe this book is a good introduction to the diagnosis of BPD for students and beginning mental health professionals. For these readers, we have provided an appendix that offers a fuller discussion of more advanced theoretical and technical matters.

We also wrote this book to share with you that there are new reasons to hope! In only the past ten years, several large, comprehensive research projects have studied groups of individuals with a diagnosis of BPD over many years. These research projects were the first of their kind and have contributed enormously to the current state of knowledge. One of the first research papers to report on these studies, published in 2005, came to what at the time was a quite startling conclusion:

> After careful analysis of the first six years of [this study, it was found] that remissions [patient getting completely better] are far more common than previously recognized . . . These remissions are quite stable and thus, recurrences are quite rare . . . It was also found that borderline patients were improving [in their relationships] over time . . . [and that the] functioning of remitted patients continued to improve as time progressed. *Taken together, these results suggest that the prognosis for BPD is better than previously recognized* [emphasis added].[1]

Borderline personality disorder is a psychiatric diagnosis that has been difficult to comprehend almost since it was first described in the late 1930s. As the decades have gone by, it has continued to be controversial. Experts still disagree on how to define it, diagnose it, and best treat those who have BPD. One expert described persons who have borderline personality disorder as "the psychological equivalent of third degree burn patients."[2] This apt description captures how impaired and fragile these individuals often are, how difficult it can be to fully grasp the complexity and range of their problems, and how challenging it can be to successfully treat them. Many introductory books about this diagnosis, and most books for general readers, skirt these complexities and uncertainties. They confidently quote the diagnostic criteria of the DSM (the American Psychiatric Association's *Diagnostic and Statistical Manual of Mental Disorders*) in an attempt to provide simple and straightforward answers to questions about borderline personality. This is not such a book.

We recommend that you set aside any idea that you will be able to breeze through this book in an evening or two and come away with a full understanding of this diagnosis and its treatment. There is an old adage that goes something like this: "Every complex question has a simple answer—and it's always wrong." We believe that this applies more to borderline personality disorder than to any other psychiatric diagnosis.

Therefore, in writing this book, we have decided that we're not going to take any shortcuts, that we won't avoid what may seem like merely theoretical discussions if they are important to understanding these problems better. We will dive into the scientific literature feet first and explain its implications (providing complete scholarly references for those who feel up to wrestling with the original research papers as well).

For example, we believe that you can't grasp what a personality disorder is unless you have some idea of what "personality" is, so we have devoted an entire chapter to this topic.

Individuals who receive a diagnosis of borderline personality disorder are often prescribed antidepressant medication or mood-stabilizer medication. Thus, it's important to know something about the group of illnesses that psychiatrists call "mood disorders."

One of the most successful types of psychotherapy ("talk therapy") for people with borderline personality disorder is called *dialectical behavioral therapy* (DBT for short). We are going to spend some time defining and talking about "behavior" as psychologists think about it and about "behavioral therapy" as well, because we believe this will enhance your understanding of the borderline diagnosis.

With this book, then, you are going to get a crash course in psychology and psychiatry. It may be slow going for a while, but we think your effort and patience will pay off with a knowledge of these problems that will be deep as well as broad.

For all these reasons, we recommend that you resist any temptation to dip into the treatment chapters before reading the beginning sections, where we provide the background necessary to understand the condition and how treatments are chosen. Perhaps more than for any other psychiatric condition, treatment for borderline personality disorder is never "one size fits all." Every person is unique in the combination of difficulties, and therefore, every treatment plan is unique.

We recognize how difficult this will be to do. Persons with this diagnosis engender strong feelings—anger, frustration, bewilderment, fear—in those around them. They have a tendency to provoke crises in their relationships and environments, and it can seem as if the whirlwind of problems and emergencies that swirls around them never ends.

But we believe it is absolutely necessary to approach the problems that persons with this diagnosis have by taking a step backward, to get out of the "crisis mode" that any recent emergency has set off and instead explore all the different aspects of this disorder objectively, thoroughly, and, yes, slowly and deliberately.

Trainees in psychiatry, psychology, and other mental health professions quickly learn the importance of not letting their patients' problems and behaviors provoke them into reacting emotionally. Although this is profoundly challenging when the "patient" is you or someone you care about, we hope that knowledge and understanding will provide a valuable buffer against unhelpful emotional reactions.

ALTHOUGH THE WORD *borderline* as applied to a psychiatric condition did not appear in print until 1938, this condition has existed for at least as long as writers have recorded human personality and behaviors.

Among the Greek myths, scholars point to the sea nymph Calypso from Homer's *Odyssey* as embodying some of the qualities of a person who has borderline personality disorder. Calypso rescued Odysseus when he washed up half dead on her island home and nursed him back to health, but she was so threatened by the thought that he would then leave her that she imprisoned him in a cave for three years. Persons who have borderline personality disorder have a desperate need for nurturing that seems insatiable and can be so consuming and smothering to those around them that they end up losing exactly what they crave most: caring relationships.

Mary Todd Lincoln, the wife of Abraham Lincoln, had severe problems with depression, was impulsive and unpredictable in her conduct, and was famous for furious outbursts whenever she was thwarted in even the most trivial ways. While she was first lady, she was convinced that those in Washington society hated her and were spreading lies about her. By the time she left the White House, she had completely alienated her entire family. Her only surviving son, Robert, spent much of his adult life estranged from her, getting involved with her affairs in her old age only when she was increasingly unstable and nearly homeless—and then to help arrange for her commitment to an asylum. All these facts are quite consistent with a diagnosis of borderline personality disorder.

In our own time, Diana, Princess of Wales, wrote of her struggles with loneliness, depression, and fear of being abandoned. She grew up in a troubled household, often with one or both parents absent or emotionally preoccupied. She had such painful self-doubt that she wept before and after speaking engagements. She developed an eating disorder and engaged in self-destructive behaviors, including cutting and several suicide attempts.[3,4] All of these facts support a diagnosis of borderline personality disorder, though no one, of course, can say for sure whether she had BPD. Despite her troubles, however, Diana was a caring and loving mother, a woman who demonstrated an ability to instantly and warmly connect with people, a sincere compassion for the sick and the outcast, and an unlimited desire to make the world a better place. Despite any personality disorder she may have had, she was so widely loved that her tragic death resulted in widespread feelings of shock and loss marked by mourning all over the world.

We could add many other names to this list, names that you would instantly recognize, not because of their struggles with a potentially devastating psychiatric disorder but because of their great accomplishments in fields as divergent as literature, the arts, and politics.

WE THINK THAT YOU will find this book not only informative but encouraging and reassuring. We hope you will return to it in whatever journey you are about to take, whether that journey is toward a goal of recovery from borderline personality disorder, toward a fuller and more empathetic understanding of it, or toward becoming a helping professional for persons who have this complicated and often misunderstood disorder.

Understanding
the Problem

CHAPTER 1

The Clinical Picture

Borderline personality disorder is a whirling, tumultuous collection of painful feelings, stormy relationships, confused thinking, and desperate destructive (and self-destructive) behaviors. Few other groups of people are so tormented, and so tormenting to those who love them.

Their problems are so numerous, varied, and complex that it will take us many pages in this book to disentangle them enough to provide any explanation for them. In this chapter, we don't try just yet to explain anything, but simply describe the collection of problems that would result in a person receiving this still controversial psychiatric diagnosis.

ANNE'S VOICE WAS SO INDISTINCT *that Peter thought maybe the phone wasn't working properly.*

"I think . . . I think you better come over."

"Anne, where are you? Are you at home?"

"Umm . . . I'm, umm . . . I'm here all by myself." She sounded groggy —or drunk.

"Anne, have you started drinking again already?"

"Umm . . . OK."

The line went dead.

"Anne? Anne?"

The only sound was a dial tone.

"I can't believe it," Peter thought, and then, "Not again, she's not going to do this to me again." Peter turned off his cell phone and set it down smartly on the kitchen table before walking through the living room and into his office. He sat down at his computer and opened the Web site he was

working on. *The lines of computer code stared back from the screen, but he couldn't focus on them.*

He walked back to the kitchen, picked up the cell phone, and turned it on as he went back to his desk. He sat down again. His eyes wandered from the computer screen to the phone and back again. He tried to focus on the lines of code. "She'll call back if she really needs me." But it was no use; he picked up the phone and pressed the call button. He felt his heart pounding with fear and anger as it rang; no one answered, and he heard Anne's voicemail greeting: "I can't talk to you now because I'm doing something totally fabulous that I couldn't possibly interrupt. Leave me a message."

As he drove toward downtown, Peter thought back on the past year. He had met Anne at an opening reception at the art gallery that had mounted a show of his photography. She had sought him out in the crowded gallery, throwing her arm around him as if they were fast friends rather than complete strangers.

"This is the first time I've seen your work, and I'm already your biggest fan," she'd announced by way of introduction.

Before Peter knew it, they were talking every day. Anne was nearly twenty years older than Peter, who was a new art institute graduate doing freelance Web design to support himself while trying to launch a photojournalism career. She had insisted on getting his phone number that night and had called him the next day offering to introduce him to a friend of hers who worked for the newspaper. Over the ensuing weeks, she'd invited him to accompany her to private art shows and exclusive museum previews. They'd talk for hours about photography and art. It wasn't anything romantic, he would explain to his girlfriend (on what seemed like a weekly basis). "She's only a friend, more like a patron. I'd never be able to connect with the people she introduces me to on my own." Not that Anne hadn't had more than her fair share of romance. Peter had lost track of the number of ex-lovers she had mentioned to him.

That was when he first started to get uncomfortable. There was just something about the way she would share so many intimate details about herself with him, a younger man she had just met, that wasn't . . . well, appropriate. He couldn't put his finger on it, but it just didn't seem right. When Anne began to call because she needed "someone to talk to" about problems, he became even more uncomfortable. Peter began to realize that Anne was not what he had thought her to be: a mature, sophisticated woman who was vivacious and witty, someone with mutual interests who offered nuanced opinions and professional opportunities. Instead, the tables had turned, and she seemed to now depend on him emotionally.

Peter also started to realize that she drank too much and now knew that she had been involved in some pretty tumultuous relationships. He remembered the chill he had felt when she told him that one of her former boyfriends had taken out a restraining order against her. "He deserved what he got," she had said. It had been the most angry he had ever seen her. "I should have killed him," she'd screamed, then said in a completely calm voice, "I don't know why he freaked out; the insurance company paid for his goddamn car." Peter didn't ask for details, just as he hadn't when she had told him about her psychiatric hospitalizations.

It had been right after that conversation that Peter had decided he needed to put more distance between himself and Anne, maybe not return her phone calls quite so promptly—but that's when the problems really started. It was as if she sensed the change immediately, as if she had some ultrasensitive emotional radar that sounded the alarm the moment it detected the slightest pull-back on Peter's part. She'd leave tearful messages accusing him of ignoring her if he waited until the next day to return a phone call. The more Peter tried to set some limits, the more desperate she seemed to become. Then the tearfulness turned into accusations. "You're trying to drive me crazy," she'd said, slurring her words, in one 2 a.m. message. "You're doing this to me to put me back in the crazy house. Why do you hate me?" and then, "What do you want me to do, kill myself?"

Peter felt trapped. How had this happened? How had he been drawn into this? What might she do to herself? He had rushed out of his apartment that night and driven to Anne's condominium. There was no answer when he knocked on her door, and after some hesitation, he used the key that she had insisted on giving him, now realizing that this was probably what she had meant when she'd said she wanted him to have one "just in case there's an emergency." He called her name from the entryway and noticed movement on the living room couch; there was an empty bottle of vodka on an end table. Anne had evidently drunk herself to sleep on the couch. He

helped her rouse herself and get into the bedroom. "I'm fine . . . I'm fine,"
she murmured as she climbed into bed.

That had been a month ago, and now he found himself in the same situation.
Just like before, it had been nearly midnight when Anne had called, slurring
her words, nearly incoherent, and then hanging up on him before he could
fully assess what was going on with her. She'd given him just enough infor-
mation to make him worry about her, but had cut off communication as
soon as he started trying to help. She seemed to do this again and again in
their relationship. Every interaction felt like a tug-of-war now.

Peter knew she had bottles and bottles of pills in her medicine cabinet.
She'd told him she'd lied to her psychiatrist about getting rid of them. He
remembered the conversation quite clearly now. "I want to keep them just
in case," she'd told Peter.

"In case what?" he'd asked.

"Oh, just in case," she'd said slyly. He simply didn't know how to re-
spond to this sort of thing. On the one hand, Peter knew he was being
manipulated; but he also knew Anne was "sick" in some way he didn't
understand and that he would feel horrible if something really bad hap-
pened. He wanted to help her, but the more he tried, the worse she seemed
to feel. Anger mixed with guilt, concern with contempt. No show of con-
cern or support from him was ever sufficient; rather, she'd raise the stakes
with some new crisis of neediness—like tonight's—demanding more and
more from him. She was an emotional black hole, sucking everything out of
him. Why would anyone do that?

This story illustrates many of the kinds of problems that are usually
seen in someone with the diagnosis of borderline personality disorder.
The account is seriously deficient, however, in one important way: it
doesn't say much about how people who receive this diagnosis feel "on
the inside." These excerpts from several first-person accounts of what it
feels like will give you some idea:

My moods were consistently erratic. I was angry, hostile, sad, guilty,
depressed, functional, angry, hostile, sad, and depressed . . . I was

trapped in this tunnel of good and bad, angelic and evil, righteous and sinful, intolerable and commendable. I searched for a way to combine the two polarities and found no way. I would go from happy loving adoration of my new dog to condemnable hate. In seconds.[1]

"I'm horrible," I told the man on the other end of the [suicide hotline]. "I hate myself. I'm crazy." It would really surprise him that once upon a time I used to be somebody. People who knew me, I told him, wouldn't believe that all this was going on. They think I'm a nice person. *They don't know me.*[2]

It is nearly impossible for me to form friendships. On the other hand, once I do form a relationship, it becomes the most important thing in my life . . . It has been said that there is no gray area in a borderline's relationships . . . that borderline people forget the friendship when the friend is gone, forget they are loved when the lover is gone. Borderlines don't really know how to *miss* somebody. Life in general and people in particular always seem markedly temporary.[3]

Three weeks ago I dug one of my holes so deep, I thought I might not make it out intact. I was in such conflicting darkness that my eyes could barely distinguish any light. When I dove in, I forgot to bring my tools. My flashlight. My shovel. I simply dug and dug with raw, aching fingers. And this is where I remained. Time passed so slowly, I was unable to calculate just how long I had been underground. Nothing sustained like the darkness I felt. I withdrew from reality and sat in a quiet numbness that only one suffering this affliction can feel. I mourned. I grieved. I panicked. Yet these feelings seemed to pass in front of me in those shadows. I was unable to feel anything but my own self-pity. My emotions so raw that I worried that I may bleed to death. I was a product of my own rigorous self-deprecation. Constantly berating myself for feeling so deeply.[4]

For me having borderline personality disorder is having constant and unremitting feelings of unbearable and overwhelming sadness, anger, depression, negativity, hatred, emptiness, frustration, helplessness, passivity, procrastination, loneliness and boredom. Feelings of anxiety are like silent screams in my head and it is as if masses of electricity are channeling through my body.[5]

These passages make an extremely important point about this diagnosis: the misery that persons with this diagnosis cause for others is nothing compared to the misery that *they* feel. It's difficult for those close to the person with these problems to understand this, but as with many psychiatric problems, drawing what seem to be logical conclusions about the situation can lead one astray. This bears further explanation.

When someone seems to intentionally behave in such a way as to make you uncomfortable or angry or scared, it's natural to assume that they are doing so out of maliciousness. We'll define that word to make this point more clearly. The *Oxford English Dictionary* defines malicious intent as "The intention or desire to do evil or cause injury to another person; active ill will or hatred . . . the desire to discomfort." For persons with a borderline diagnosis, however, this is usually not true. Rather, they behave as they do as a desperate attempt to assuage the terrible feelings that the passages above illustrate. The dilemma for someone who has BPD is that she is full of terrible and uncontrollable emotions but doesn't have the coping skills necessary to feel better in any other way. This gets to the heart of what the term *personality disorder* means, and we will discuss this at greater length in the next chapter. For now, however, we will flesh out our description of these problems.

Features of the Borderline Diagnosis

In focusing on the features of this diagnosis, a reasonable starting point is the *Diagnostic and Statistical Manual of Mental Disorders* (DSM).*
The DSM began as a list of the features of psychiatric illnesses to assist researchers. It was compiled by experts on mental illnesses to make

---

*This discussion is based on the edition of the DSM that is current as of this writing, the DSM-IV (fourth edition). A new edition is now being developed and is scheduled to be published in the spring of 2013.

Table 1.1 Borderline personality disorder in the DSM

1. Problems with emotional control and modulation
   a. Instability of mood
   b. Intense and difficult-to-control anger
   c. Impulsivity in areas that are potentially self-damaging (substance abuse, sexual behaviors)

2. Damaged self-identity
   a. Unstable image of self
   b. Long-term feelings of emptiness and frantic efforts to avoid real or imagined abandonment
   c. Short-lived periods of feeling paranoid or "in a trance"

3. Behavioral consequences of (1) and (2)
   a. Unstable and intense interpersonal relationships
   b. Recurrent suicidal behavior: suicide attempts or threats, or self-mutilating behaviors, such as cutting

Source: Adapted from American Psychiatric Association, Task Force on DSM-IV. *Diagnostic and Statistical Manual of Mental Disorders: DSM-IV-TR*, 4th text revision ed. (Washington, D.C.: American Psychiatric Association, 2000).

it easier for researchers to agree on who does and who doesn't have a particular disorder in order to do consistent work. If a dozen different researchers are doing research on the treatment of schizophrenia, it's obviously extremely important that they all use the same methods to diagnose the illness. The DSM was originally developed for exactly this purpose. Unfortunately, the DSM has come to be used for all kinds of other purposes for which it was not originally intended. For example, it is often thought of as the ultimate authority in diagnosis. This has created many problems—but that's another story. For our purpose here, a good starting point is to provide a list of the features of people diagnosed with BPD, the DSM diagnostic criteria, developed by professionals who specialize in treating these patients and who have thought long and hard about their problems. In table 1.1, and in the following paragraphs, we have rephrased and rearranged the DSM diagnostic criteria to make them easier to understand.

Problems with emotional control and modulation. These individuals have constantly shifting emotions that they have great difficulty controlling.

Their moods are constantly changing, and they feel continually buffeted by strong emotions, like a small boat sailing through high winds and choppy waters. They repeatedly lose control of their feelings, especially negative feelings, but also positive ones. They fly into rages at the least provocation, responding with anger that is unexpected and completely out of proportion to what would be appropriate to the situation. Their romantic attachments develop rapidly and quickly become intense and all-consuming.

Usually, as people mature, we become better and better at getting a hold on our emotions whenever we realize that not doing so will cause problems for us. If your boss says something that makes you angry, you simply don't allow yourself to lose your temper and start yelling. "She made me really mad, but I just bit my tongue" captures this idea. Individuals with borderline personality disorder, however, have a great deal of difficulty doing this.

Their inability to damp down emotions also means that people with a borderline diagnosis can be carried away on their emotional waves into potentially self-destructive behaviors. Because they cannot rein in their emotions, they cannot rein in their behavior. This may involve pleasurable behaviors—sexual behaviors, drinking too much, driving too fast—or desperate attempts to stop experiencing negative feelings—going on spending sprees, using drugs, binging on food.

Damaged self-identity. This is considered by many experts to be the central problem for persons with the borderline diagnosis. The exact wording in the DSM is "identity disturbance," but this fails to capture the severity of the emptiness, worthlessness, and aloneness that they feel. One of us had a colleague who would describe persons with the borderline diagnosis as "having a black hole where most of us have a sense of who we are." Unable to feel good about themselves, they become clingy in relationships quickly, seeking constant attention from others as well as reassurance that they are cared about. One of the consequences of this problem is that they become frantic if they think that someone in their life might leave them. They may react by setting up increasingly high-stake situations that force others to *prove* they care. This inevitably has the opposite effect sooner or later, as they end up alienating the persons they are trying to get to show concern by making them feel manipulated and angry. When this happens, the other person becomes angry or frustrated and pulls away, or may simply say something critical, which reinforces this sense of worthlessness and emptiness and can lead in turn to self-destructive behaviors such as suicidal gestures.

The problems with sense of self can be so severe that these individuals begin to have distortions in their thinking or even begin to lose touch with reality. They may become convinced that they are being singled out for mistreatment or may otherwise misinterpret what others say or do. Feeling "out of control" or "crazy" is common, and some of these individuals seem to almost get lost in themselves at times, in a trancelike state that psychiatrists call *dissociation*, which we discuss in chapter 7 in more detail.

Behavioral consequences. The extreme moods and chronic feelings of emptiness create untold difficulties for these individuals as well as those around them.

Their intense feelings make their interpersonal relationships intense and troubled, full of turmoil and conflicts. The term *push-pull* relationship was coined to capture the strained and unstable relationships of persons with the borderline diagnosis. Those who care about someone who has BPD feel alternately pushed away and pulled in by her, alternately seduced, manipulated, and even coerced.

The emotional features of the borderline diagnosis make recurrent suicidal behaviors extremely common. Feeling chronically empty and worthless, experiencing extremes of emotions, and being impulsive are a certain recipe for these behaviors. They frequently take the form of what psychiatrists call *suicidal gestures*. These are attempts at self-harm that are unlikely to cause death, but rather seem to be intended to send someone a message. They can usually be better understood as seeking attention and nurturing from others, or seeking to demonstrate the depth of the individual's emotional despair.

Self-mutilating behaviors such as cutting can sometimes also be viewed in a slightly different way than people might assume. Some individuals with the borderline diagnosis will say that they cut on their body to "keep from feeling numb" or "just to make all the bad feelings stop." Drug use or binge-eating behaviors often stem from similar motivations. One of our patients stated that she became emaciated from refusing to eat "so that I look on the outside how I feel on the inside."

Distortions of thinking. In some persons with the diagnosis, distortions of thinking may be so extreme that they border on the psychotic symptoms of severe mental illnesses like schizophrenia.

> I feel unloved and unlovable and constantly doubt that anyone likes me or even knows I exist. Both my body and mind feel like they are toxic and polluted. I always feel dirty and scruffy no matter how many baths I take. My sense of physical self is constantly changing—I am not sure what I look like and my facial features keep changing shape and getting uglier and uglier. Mirrors are terrifying—I always think I'm fatter or skinnier than I am.
>
> Sometimes it seems like people are sneering and laughing at me all the time and attractive women look at me like they are murdering me with their eyes. Other times it is as if I am invisible. At times I hate everyone and everything. Ideas about who I am and what I want to do fluctuate from week to week. My perspectives, thoughts and decisions are easily undermined by what other people think or say and I often put on different voices to fit in. I am never satisfied with my appearance, but then I am never satisfied *per se*—perfect is not even perfect enough.[5]

These distortions of thinking, which frequently occur in the setting of severe emotional crises, contributed to the origin of the term *borderline* for this disorder, because they suggested that these patients had a condition that was on the borderline between personality disorders and psychotic illnesses such as schizophrenia. We now believe that no such relationship exists and that this is not a helpful way of thinking about the disorder, but unfortunately the term *borderline personality* has become so entrenched in the psychiatric literature that it continues to be the term that we use. Many people with the borderline diagnosis never have these symptoms, but those who do are understandably terrified by them. Also, because the symptoms can be so dramatic, they can overshadow the more subtle symptoms inherent to the borderline syndrome and occasionally lead to misdiagnosis.

Although the DSM criteria are helpful, they miss, or at least underestimate, several key symptoms and issues that these individuals face. A more complete picture emerges when one considers other types of problems, specifically, the typical ways in which these individuals cope. Two psychologists, Drs. Jonathon Shedler and Drew Westen, have developed a way of diagnosing personality disorders that involves asking a clinician who is treating a patient and who has therefore spent many hours with him to read through a list of 200 different symptoms and ways of coping that people may have and decide which statements describe their patient really well, not so well, or not at all.[6] An experienced therapist who knows her patient well can easily decide if the statement that her patient "appears to want to 'punish' himself/herself by creating situations that lead to unhappiness" is accurate, or whether the patient "tends to blame others for his/her own failures or shortcomings; tends to believe his/her problems are caused by external factors." Another feature of this procedure is that it allows the clinician to decide whether the patient has relevant personal strengths. For example, one of the statements is "He/she can assert himself/herself effectively and appropriately when necessary."

This procedure, called the Shedler-Westen Assessment Procedure, or SWAP, allows a much more detailed and complete picture of the individual to be painted than the dozen or so "diagnostic criteria" of the DSM. When these researchers asked over one hundred experienced psychiatrists and psychologists to use this technique to assess a patient of theirs whom they were treating for borderline personality, quite a few other aspects of these patients emerged that the DSM only hints at—or leaves out entirely (see table 1.2). In fact, the three top attributes these clinicians selected as describing their patients who had BPD aren't even among the DSM criteria.

The most striking of these is the multitude of bad feelings these individuals are constantly struggling with: depression, anxiety, helplessness, feelings of inferiority and of being an outcast. The authors of the study concluded that "DSM-IV may understate the . . . pain that

Table 1.2 Items from the Shedler-Westen Assessment Procedure-200 selected by therapists as describing their patients who have borderline personality disorder, listed in rank order

Tends to feel unhappy, depressed, or despondent

Emotions tend to spiral out of control, leading to extremes of anxiety, sadness, rage, excitement, etc.

Is unable to soothe or comfort self when distressed; requires involvement of another person to help regulate affect

Tends to be anxious

Tends to feel she/he is inadequate, mistreated, or victimized

Tends to become irrational when strong emotions are stirred up; may show a noticeable decline from customary level of functioning

Tends to be overly needy or dependent; requires excessive reassurance or approval

Tends to "catastrophize"; is prone to see problems as disastrous, insolvable, etc.

Tends to feel helpless, powerless, or at the mercy of forces outside his/her control

Tends to feel like an outcast or outsider; feels as if she/he does not truly belong

Note: The first item was used the most often to describe patients, the second item the second most often used, etc.

borderline personality disorder patients feel."[7] They also concluded that "negative affect," a psychiatric term for depression and anxiety, is "central" to the disorder. Another term for this swirl of uncomfortable feelings is *dysphoria*. We will come back to this issue of chronic negative emotions in a later chapter when we discuss the treatment for depression and anxiety with medications. Obviously, an individual with this problem will not improve unless these uncomfortable feelings, especially depression, are addressed.

Another aspect that emerged from this study is the individual's *inability to self-soothe* when upset; this means that they are driven to obtain this soothing and comfort from others. This goes a long way to explain the tendency of these individuals to get into intense relationships quickly and to be sensitive and react strongly to any perceived pull-back in relationships. In the next section, we will talk about more of the features of the borderline condition derived from this work and then combine them with the DSM criteria to provide a fairly complete clinical picture of these individuals.

Making the Diagnosis of Borderline Personality Disorder

We hope that the last section makes clear that borderline personality disorder is a complex problem with many different features. These features include:

- negative and unpleasant internal emotions and feelings, or as psychiatrists and psychologists say, negative "affective experiences"
- a damaged sense of self and chronic feelings of inferiority and emptiness
- an inability to cope with and modulate or rein in these inner experiences
- the behavioral problems that result from the first three

We've tried to capture the big picture in table 1.3.

Perhaps most significant is the ever-present swirl of various painful, *uncomfortable emotions*. From simple unhappiness to what Pulitzer Prize–winning author William Styron called the "brown-out" of depression, to abject hopelessness and despair, people who have BPD struggle with down feelings day after day, month after month. Anxiety is often a part of this picture, as is what one of our patients called the "black energy" of hostility and irritability.

Another aspect of the condition is that the chronic dysphoric feelings are accompanied in these individuals by what can be understood as a *damaged sense of self*. They suffer from profound feelings of inadequacy, inferiority, and failure as well as feelings of emptiness and boredom. This damaged sense of self can also be seen in many persons who have serious depression. Serious depression has a peculiar way of distorting the way we feel about ourselves that diseases of the body do not. As one of our professors said, "When a person has a toothache, he doesn't start to think that he *is* the toothache." But when a person is se-

Table 1.3 Features of borderline personality disorder

Almost always full of painful, uncomfortable emotions
    Unhappiness, depression, or despondency
    Anxiety
    Anger and hostility

Inability to regulate emotions
    Has emotions that change rapidly and unpredictably
    Tends to spiral out of control emotionally, which leads to extremes of anxiety, sadness, rage, excitement
    Unable to soothe or comfort self when distressed; requires involvement of another person to help regulate emotions
    Tends to "catastrophize"; is prone to see problems as disastrous and insolvable
    Becomes attached quickly or intensely; develops feelings and expectations of others that are not warranted by the history or context of the relationship
    Tends to feel she/he will be rejected or abandoned by those who are emotionally significant
    Tends to feel misunderstood, mistreated, or victimized
    Tends to become irrational when strong emotions are stirred up and shows a decline from usual level of functioning
    Tends to act impulsively, without regard for consequences
    Is simultaneously needy of and rejecting toward others (craves intimacy and caring, but tends to reject it when offered)
    Has interpersonal relationships that tend to be unstable, chaotic, and rapidly changing

Damaged sense of self
    Lacks a stable image of who she/he is or would like to become: attitudes, values, goals, and feelings about self may be unstable and changing
    Feels inadequate, inferior, like a failure
    Tends to feel emptiness and boredom
    Tends to feel helpless, powerless, at the mercy of forces outside his/her control
    Feels like an outcast or outsider, as if he/she does not truly belong
    Tends to be overly needy or dependent; requires excessive reassurance or approval

riously depressed, he often starts to attribute his bad feelings to who he "really is" or to something he has done (or not done). Persons who have BPD seem especially prone to this problem, even during times when their depression is not so severe. Recognizing that the way they feel most of the time is different from what they see in those around them, they feel like outcasts or outsiders, as if they do not truly belong. Their view of their future is affected too, and they often lack a stable image of who they are or would like to become. Their attitudes, values, goals, and feelings about who they are is often unstable and changing. It's not difficult to see how the combination of chronic negative emotions and a damaged sense of self can lead to a tendency for the person who has BPD to feel helpless, powerless, and at the mercy of forces outside her control.

Many persons who have serious mood disorders such as major depression struggle over long periods with uncomfortable feelings. What makes the uncomfortable feelings so much more difficult for a person who has BPD is that she is far less equipped to cope with them and much less able to modulate them or keep them from taking over. The emotions of these individuals change rapidly and unpredictably and easily spiral out of control, leading to extremes of anxiety, sadness, rage, or excitement. They can go from mildly irritated to utterly enraged in a heartbeat, or from feeling merely disappointed to suicidal just as quickly. They cannot talk themselves out of these spirals but tend to "catastrophize"; that is, they immediately imagine the worst-case scenario in every situation and see every problem as disastrous and insolvable. When strong emotions are stirred up, they can become irrational and show a decline from their usual level of functioning.

Lacking the capacity to soothe or comfort themselves when distressed, they need others to help them regulate emotions. This means they require constant reassurance and approval and are often extremely needy or dependent in relationships. They become attached to others quickly and often intensely, developing feelings and expectations of others that are not warranted. This can easily lead to feeling misunderstood, mistreated, or victimized when, inevitably, someone around them proves unwilling or unable to help them in some way. It doesn't take too many of these experiences for them to expect that they will sooner or later be rejected or abandoned by those who are emotionally significant. Another aspect of this feature is they are often simultaneously needy of and rejecting toward others, craving intimacy and caring, but tending to rebuff it for fear of being rejected first. Thus, their interpersonal relationships tend to be unstable, chaotic, and rapidly changing.

We want to make it clear at this point that this problem is not easy to diagnose and that the diagnosis does not necessarily point to a particular treatment or set of treatments. As you will see in later chapters, several psychiatric problems share many of the features of this diagnosis, and it can be fiendishly difficult to tell the difference between them. Only an experienced clinician can make this diagnosis and then only after getting to know the patient quite well. One of us trained with a professor of psychiatry who warned that it was impossible to make a diagnosis of a personality disorder until one had treated the patient for at least six months. That may be a bit of an exaggeration but makes a good point: even the most experienced therapist cannot make sound judgments about a problem that includes subtleties of personality as well as symptoms that are shared by many other disorders without really getting to know his patient well.

The Borderline Conundrum

It's not difficult to see how the various aspects of this disorder reinforce each other and make it almost impossible for persons who have BPD to deal with their various problems on their own.

As an example, the tendency of individuals who have BPD to feel strong uncontrollable emotions may lead them to start using alcohol or drugs as a way to dull these emotions, which may lead them to see themselves as alcoholics or addicts, thus reinforcing their already damaged sense of self. They may seek another person to help them feel better about themselves, a friend or a therapist. But they are likely to become clingy and demanding toward this other person because of their inability to manage strong emotions and soothe uncomfortable feelings on their own. When the other person inevitably tries to set some limits on the clinginess, this triggers more strong emotions in persons who have BPD, which may lead to an increase in their use of alcohol or drugs, which in turn leads to . . . well, you get the idea. When these individuals experience unmanageable bad feelings, they reach for some solution outside themselves, leading to unhealthy one-sided relationships or self-destructive behaviors, which cause more bad feelings and increasingly dramatic self-destructive "cries for help": binges of various sorts, cutting behaviors, suicidal threats or even attempts. The borderline conundrum is that attempts to make things better usually end up making things worse, leading to increasingly desperate attempts that make everything increasingly worse. Therapists who treat patients with borderline disorder are familiar with these vicious cycles and know how difficult it can be to interrupt them. Sometimes the only way to do so involves psychiatric hospitalization—which again reinforces that individual's perception of himself as a failure and an outcast—but where at least there is an army of professionals available 24/7 to help him deal with the storms of emotions.

These problems may appear impossible to solve. Indeed, the way they all seem to trigger and reinforce each other, with the usual solutions often making things worse rather than better, might lead to a lot of pessimism. Fortunately, they are not insolvable. However, as we hope we've made clear, the borderline diagnosis contains multifaceted sets of difficulties for which there are no easy answers. Knowing how to start making things better requires "unpacking" these many and intertwined problems and understanding them and their interrelationships before one can know where to start. The DSM is woefully inadequate for this endeavor. Instead, in chapter 3, we will use a method developed at Johns Hopkins that allows for a much richer comprehension of psychiatric problems and provides straightforward advice on what the best treatments should be.

CHAPTER 2

"Personality" and More

Understanding "Personality"

Everybody has a personality, and no two are exactly alike. We use all kinds of words to talk about people's personalities and to describe people to each other. "I can see why Susan is a good nurse; she's such a *caring* person." "I'm not sure about asking Mike to join us on the project team; he's so *unpredictable*." "I can see Maggie turning out to be a great entrepreneur; she's got such a *bold* streak and is a real *risk taker*." "I'm sure we can count on Phil to be here; he's such a *dependable* guy." In fact, one of the most frequently used psychological tests to measure aspects of personality was derived from a sophisticated analysis of just such words.

Obviously, it would not be necessary to have so many words to talk about personality if everyone's personalities were similar. Take, for example, the descriptor *dependable*. Think about half a dozen or so friends and acquaintances. Who are "more dependable" and who are "less dependable" people? Odds are you can rank them in "dependability order," something that is possible only because they all vary in their dependability. Quite possibly, they vary widely; you might be comfortable asking several among them for a ride to a party but would trust only one of them to get you to an important appointment on time. Undoubtedly, you can also rank them according to the other qualities mentioned above. Who among them is the most *caring*? The most *unpredictable*? Psychologists call these qualities *traits*, and the branch of psychology that is interested in personality has worked over many years to understand them better.

Another reason this ranking process is possible is that in your interactions with these folks over time, you have discovered that many aspects of their personalities don't change much from one day to the next, or even year to year. This is perhaps the most essential aspect of personality: it is an *enduring* aspect of a person, something that tends not to change much over time. Our personality doesn't depend on the situation we're in or who we're with. A person brings his personality with him to all aspects of life, whether at work or at play, and to all his relationships, with family and friends and lovers (and car rental agents and waiters in restaurants and—well, you get the idea). One psychology textbook defines personality as the "organized set of characteristics possessed by a person that uniquely influences his or her cognitions [thinking patterns], motivations, and behaviors in various situations."[1]

The *Diagnostic and Statistical Manual* (DSM) of the American Psychiatric Association says pretty much the same thing, defining personality as "enduring patterns of perceiving, relating to, and thinking about the environment and oneself that are exhibited in a wide range of social and personal contexts." Put more simply, our personality is who we are: how we think about ourselves, about others, and about the world influences the way we act no matter where or when. As the great German psychiatrist-turned-philosopher Karl Jaspers said in 1913, "We see personality in the particular way an individual expresses himself, in the way he moves, how he experiences and reacts to situations, how he loves, grows jealous, how he conducts his life in general, what needs he has, what are his longings and aims, what are his ideals and how he shapes them, what values guide him and what he does, what he creates and how he acts."[2]

A fundamental aspect of personality is that it appears to be intrinsic, seemingly inborn, or at the least apparent from a very young age. If you've ever had a mom proudly show off her new baby to you, one of the things she may tell you is that "this baby has such a different personality from my first." Perhaps you're a parent who has noticed this in your own children. Even before they can talk, some babies are more easily soothed than others, or more "fussy," more or less curious or energetic. A considerable body of research has confirmed that substantial differences in personality traits can be identified even in very young children.

In 1956, several child psychiatrists at New York University embarked on an ambitious research project to evaluate personality in 136 children, following them from infancy through toddlerhood and early childhood over 10 years. (They used the term "temperament" rather than "personality," but the idea is similar.) By asking parents to report on their child's behaviors, observing the children as they attended nursery school, interviewing their teachers, and meeting with the children and their mothers and observing their interactions, as well as by assessing the children with psychological tests, the researchers collected enormous amounts of data. In infancy, the children were rated on things like their usual activity level, how regular they were in their sleeping and eating patterns, how they reacted to new situations (with curiosity or withdrawal), the intensity of their emotional reactions, as well as several other features of emotional life, including "quality of mood," which was described as "the amount of pleasant, joyful, friendly behavior as contrasted with unpleasant, crying and unfriendly behavior" that was typical of the child.[3]

The results were remarkable. The researchers found that important aspects of personality were apparent by the age of two, and several different groups of children could be delineated: "difficult" children, "easy" children, and those who were "slow to warm up." The difficult children had erratic sleeping and eating patterns; they tended to withdraw from new situations rather than be curious, to be slow to adapt to changes in the environment, and to be more intense and negative in their emotional reactions. About 10 percent of the total group fell into this category. The "easy" children showed an opposite pattern, being "predominantly positive in mood, highly regular [in sleeping and eating patterns], low or mild in the intensity of their reactions, rapidly adaptable, and unusually positive in their approaches to new situations." The "slow to warm up" children, as you might guess, tended to be slow to adapt to and more reluctant to engage in new situations, but they did not stand out as far as the intensity of their emotional reactions or the negativity of their moods.

Later researchers have studied how stable these qualities are over time, and again, the results are remarkable. A team in Australia who studied 450 children from infancy to 8 years found that these same personality traits show "substantial continuity over time."[4] Many other studies have also demonstrated this essential quality of personality: it is an *enduring* (but, as you will see, not necessarily a *permanent*) aspect of a person.

In the next chapter, we will discuss in more detail ways in which psychologists conceptualize personality.

What Is a Personality *Disorder*?

Think back for a moment about the persons you rated according to their dependability in the last section. Is there one on whom you would never rely for anything at all because he is so completely and repeatedly unreliable? Is there someone whose problem with dependability is so severe that he has trouble maintaining relationships, keeping a job for long, and paying bills on time? In this person, an aspect of his personality causes multiple problems in many areas of life. This is the concept behind the term *personality disorder*.

Psychotherapist scholars who have thought quite a lot about these things discuss this issue in their own diagnostic manual, the *Psychodynamic Diagnostic Manual*, where they first list the characteristics of *healthy* personality: "People [with healthy personalities] . . . can engage in satisfying relationships, can experience a relatively full range of age-expected feelings and thoughts, can function relatively flexibly when stressed . . . have a clear sense of personal identity, are well-adapted to their life circumstances, and neither experience significant distress nor impose it on others."[5]

A personality disorder is said to exist when some personality trait, or more often, a particular group of personality traits, is so extreme and so outside the range of normal that a person has problems functioning in nearly all areas of life because of it. A person's ability to develop and maintain healthy relationships with others, to function in work situations and as a member of a community, and even the ability to provide for himself is impaired; because of this, he is troubled most of the time by unhappiness, frustration, anger, and any other number of uncomfortable emotions that arise out of the situations that result from his actions. Usually, the person's personality traits also cause uncomfortable feelings in others, and this inevitably makes matters much worse:

A YOUNG POLICE OFFICER *was driving past the on-ramp to the freeway early one hot afternoon when he noticed an uncharacteristic traffic backup onto the street. He saw that a car had stopped on the ramp, blocking access to the freeway and trapping a half-dozen or so vehicles on the narrow roadway. He pulled over, but before he got out of the patrol car, he called his dispatcher. "This is Ridley in car 406 at the Brentley Street on-ramp to I-14. There's a disabled vehicle halfway up the ramp that's blocking access; better get a tow truck over here ASAP."*

As he walked up the ramp past several sweaty, exasperated motorists, Officer Ridley tried to soothe them. "It's OK, folks; tow truck's on the way; we'll get things moving in a few minutes." As he neared the disabled car, a vintage-looking Mercedes-Benz, he saw a man who looked to be in his mid-20s arguing with an older man dressed in an equally vintage-looking three-piece suit.

"What did you call me?" the younger man was shouting, "What was that? Did I hear you call me a—" He pulled back a clenched fist and was about to let loose an awful punch when Ridley grabbed his arm.

"Whoa, boys, let's settle down," said the young officer, coming between the two men.

"I offer to help this guy move his car to the side of the road and he calls me a—"

"OK, Junior, get back in your car before I arrest you for attempted assault."

"Attempted assault? What the hell kind of charge is that?"

"Go!" barked Ridley, and the young man backed off, turned around, and headed back down the ramp. "OK, sir, I'd like you to get back in your car, release the parking brake, and get ready to steer. The ramp's pretty level here." Ridley started to walk to the back of what he now saw was a quite beat-up old car. "I think I can push you to the side, and we can get some of these cars moving."

"That's not possible," said the man in the suit. "My car might get scratched if one of these idiots gets too close to it."

Ridley stopped. He slowly turned around with an incredulous look. "I'm sorry?"

"Young man, you need to stay with my car while I walk over to that gas station and bring back some gasoline."

"Now wait a minute, buddy. I'm giving the orders around here. I said—"

"Listen, you fool, I'll have you thrown off the force before you even know what happened to you. I'll call the mayor . . . and the governor and get you fired! No one is going to touch my car."

"I don't care who you're going to call," the officer said, walking up to the oddly calm man. "This car needs to move."

The police dispatcher pushed the broadcast button on the radio in front of her and spoke clearly into the microphone. "Officer calling for backup. Any available car to the Brentley Street on-ramp to I-14."

The emergency room nurse was used to having police officers in the ER, but judging from the sea of blue uniforms in front of her, it looked like half the force had just walked in.

Above a din of voices, she heard a man shouting, "You filthy pigs! You swine!" and several other more colorful words and phrases. But she was used to that too. What the man was wearing struck her as a bit unusual: a three-piece suit. "What are you bringing me, Jimmy?" she asked a burly sergeant.

"Definitely a psych case," he responded. "And we're going to stay for a while so no one gets hurt."

Several weeks later a young psychiatrist sat down and started to open a medical record on her desk. Then she stood up again. The weather had finally cooled down some over the weekend, so she opened the office window, hoping the morning air would get rid of the stuffiness in the room. A light breeze started to blow through the grimy window, and she sat down again, turning back to the folder. On the front cover, it said, "McCormick

Hospital Community Mental Health Clinic," and *"Strictly Confidential."*
She opened the folder and started to read the hospital discharge summary
on top: "This 58-year-old man was admitted to the psychiatry service from
the emergency room, where he had been brought by police after creating
a disturbance in the community." She glanced through the pages looking
for the "Hospital Course" section of the summary and noticed that the
document was much longer than usual. As she skimmed the pages, one sen-
tence caught her eye: "On the third hospital day, unbeknownst to staff, the
patient called WTMQ News and told them that he was being abused on the
unit. When the television crew arrived at the entrance to the unit, hospi-
tal administration was informed, and they in turn contacted the hospital
media relations and legal departments." She was intrigued by this, but sud-
denly the room seemed hot again. She skipped to the end of the summary.
"Primary Diagnosis: Narcissistic Personality Disorder."

She finished reading, stood up, and took a deep breath, then walked out
to a small waiting room.

"Mr. Anderson?" she said, looking around the room.

"Yes?" said an older man, looking up from a magazine. He was wear-
ing a rather worn-looking three-piece suit. "I'm Dr. Watkins," she said,
extending a hand to shake.

The man looked at her for a moment, then back down at the magazine.
"You won't do at all," he said as he casually turned the page. "I'm not talk-
ing to some rookie. Get your supervisor and bring him here at once." After
a pause, he looked up again at Dr. Watkins's rather blank face. He smiled
slightly, then looked down and turned another page. "You heard me," he
said. "What are you waiting for?"

If, while reading this story, you at some point thought, "Who does
this guy think he is?" then you already have a good grasp of what is
meant by the term personality disorder. This unfortunate man sees
himself as superior to everyone else, and this view of himself, as well
as its converse, that everyone else is inferior, causes him to treat others
in a way that causes tremendous problems for him. This story is based
on a real patient that one of us treated. Admittedly, it is somewhat of
an exaggeration—but not much. This person lived a lonely, impover-

ished, and unhappy life because his every relationship was eventually destroyed by his inability to treat anyone else as a peer, to compromise, or to be considerate of the needs and feelings of others.

The term *narcissism* comes from the Greek myth of the handsome Narcissus, who arrogantly spurned all lovers and was punished by the gods for his cruel rejection of the youth Amenias. They caused Narcissus to fall in love with his own reflection in a pool of water, and he pined away for the unobtainable lover he saw there until he died. Like Narcissus, Mr. Anderson's feelings about himself—and others—are his downfall.

This man's main difficulty, and the essence of *narcissistic personality disorder,* is well captured in the DSM-IV criteria for this diagnosis: the individual "has a grandiose sense of self-importance" and "a sense of entitlement, i.e. unreasonable expectations of especially favorable treatment or automatic compliance with his or her expectations."

It's important to point out here that everyone is narcissistic to some degree. Most people expect to be treated with respect and become angry or upset if they are not. Feeling worthy and deserving of our due is, in fact, a sign of good mental health, and too little self-esteem is a reason for concern. Of course, people vary in this trait as well; you can probably think of a friend who tends to be humble and self-effacing, or a colleague who can get a bit "full of himself" at times. Clearly, though, Mr. Anderson's self-esteem is off the charts, quite outside the range of what one usually encounters. This *extremeness* is one basis for thinking about the problem as a disorder. The other important reason for considering this a disorder is that as a result of this extremeness, this person is *impaired* in his functioning.

A third aspect of Mr. Anderson's personality might be what can be called, for lack of a better term, the *rigidity* of his personality. This aspect is emphasized in the DSM (which uses a synonym, "inflexible," instead of "rigid," but the meaning is the same). The DSM also uses the term "stable" in its criteria for the diagnosis of personality disorder. With these two terms, the DSM attempts to capture the "enduring" aspect of personality traits that we previously talked about.

One authority defines the normal flexibility in personality as being able to "look at a problem from several different angles and adopt one of several possible ways of coping with it" and suggests that a disorder is present when the person "respond[s] to stress in rigidly inflexible ways ... by relying on only one or two coping strategies ... irrespective of the situation."[5]

We now have a pretty good definition of what is meant by the term personality disorder. Someone can be said to have a personality disorder when one or several personality traits, which by definition we know to be *enduring* aspects of a person, are *extreme, inflexible,* and cause *impairment* in social, occupational, and other areas of functioning.

When Does "Personality" Become "Disorder"?

Now that we've given you a clear, concise definition of personality disorder, we're going to tell you why, as a way to think about these sorts of problems, it is imperfect at best. This is mainly because using the word *disorder* implies that one can always decide who has the problem and who doesn't. This is generally how we think about medical problems and diseases. Either you have the disorder, or you don't. Someone is either sick, or they're not.

As explained in the beginning of this chapter, however, this isn't really how personality traits work. People vary quite a bit in which of their personality traits stand out from the others and to what extent their personality traits get them into trouble (think about the dependability example again). How does one decide that a personality trait is *extreme* enough to fall into the category of a disorder? Our third standard for defining a personality disorder, *impairment,* is helpful here, but again, how does one measure and decide on impairment? Using our dependability example again, if a person's lack of dependability is just annoying to his friends, is he "impaired"? What is the threshold that should be used to put someone into the "disorder" category?

Another issue important to think about here is how a person's environment can be more or less forgiving of personality extremes and mitigate the impairment that might otherwise result from them. A rather undependable person who works in a family business run by his father is probably at lower risk of losing his job because of a tardiness problem. His lack of dependability isn't as impairing as it might be because of his particular situation. You can see how using the "impairment" ruler for deciding who does or does not have a disorder is less than perfect, too.

A more useful concept than disorders to discuss personality is *dimensions*. This idea is that, like height or weight, individuals vary widely on where they fall on the measure of various personality traits, and how likely these traits are to get them into trouble depends a lot on their environment. We will return to this important point in chapter 3, but first, just when you might have thought things were getting simpler, we're going to make it complicated again. (Welcome to psychiatry!)

Mood Disorders

It's difficult to pick up a popular magazine and not see an advertisement for one or another medication used to treat serious depression or bipolar disorder. When the antidepressant Prozac (fluoxetine) was first approved to treat serious depression in the late 1980s, it was hailed as a "revolutionary" new treatment. Really, though, it was nothing of the sort.

That's because the revolution had actually started about forty years earlier, when the natural element lithium was shown to be extremely effective in treating what was at the time called manic depression (now bipolar disorder). This was the real revolution, and it started in the 1950s. Although Prozac was a great advancement because it was far easier for people to take and vastly less toxic than earlier medications, we knew for several decades that pharmaceuticals could make the symptoms of mood disorders virtually vanish over a matter of a few weeks.

With this development, it became quite clear that there is, at some level, a chemical basis for mood. After all, if the introduction of a chemical into the body could make the symptoms go away (and pharmaceuticals are, after all, just chemicals), then depression and manic depression (bipolar disorder) must be caused by some chemistry in the body gone awry.

In ensuing decades, it has become clear that to talk about "chemistry" and "chemical imbalance" is to greatly oversimplify what underlies these problems. The focus has shifted away from chemical levels to the functioning of brain cells in one particular part of the brain (the hippocampus), but the emphasis on physical processes remains. The importance of heritability and genetics in these illnesses has also become well established, and we now know that a substantial amount of the risk for these problems is encoded in our genes. You may have noticed that we are now talking about something very different from personality—about *genes* and *brain cells* in the hippocampus and using sophisticated *chemistry* to treat these problems.

Let's look at the symptoms of mood disorders. We'll start with symptoms of the most severe type of depression, major depression, and again use the DSM diagnostic criteria as a starting point.

- Depressed mood most of the day, nearly every day, as indicated by either subjective report (feeling sad or empty) or observation made by others (appearing tearful) over a period of at least two weeks
- Markedly diminished interest or pleasure in all, or almost all, activities most of the day, nearly every day (as indicated by either subjective account or observation made by others)
- Significant weight loss when not dieting or weight gain (for example, a change of more than 5 percent of body weight in a month), or decrease or increase in appetite nearly every day
- Insomnia or sleeping too much nearly every day
- Feelings of agitation or feeling slowed down nearly every day that is significant enough to be observable by others
- Fatigue or loss of energy
- Feelings of worthlessness or excessive or inappropriate guilt (which may be delusional) nearly every day (not merely self-reproach or guilt about being sick)
- Diminished ability to think or concentrate, or indecisiveness, nearly every day (either by subjective account or as observed by others)

- Recurrent thoughts of death (not just fear of dying), recurrent suicidal thinking without a specific plan, or a suicide attempt or a specific plan for committing suicide

Reading through these symptoms should make it clear that persons with major depression are very ill. And while everyone gets down or discouraged sometimes, it's difficult to see these symptoms as bearing even a passing resemblance to that common set of feelings. One wouldn't easily mistake a person who feels depressed *almost all the time*, can't enjoy anything at all, isn't sleeping and eating properly, can't think or concentrate, has no energy, and wants to kill himself for someone who is having just a more extreme form of the "blues" that everyone gets from time to time. There is clearly a discontinuity or separation between this state of *illness* and those common feelings. Add to this observable discontinuity between major depression and normal mood the fact that *changes in brain functioning* have been observed in these individuals, that the risk for developing these problems is *inherited,* and that *pharmaceutical* interventions make them better, and clearly we are not talking about traits or dimensions that everyone shares but rather about a *disease state.*

In bipolar disorder, individuals have periods of major depression but also of elevated mood and overconfidence when they become more reckless in their behavior, as well as periods of extreme irritability such that they will shout at others or even get into fights. As with major depression, problems in brain functioning have been implicated in bipolar disorder, the risk for developing it is highly genetic, and pharmaceutical interventions are usually effective in stopping these mood fluctuations.

But now let's cycle back to the features of the borderline diagnosis. You may remember from chapter 1 that these individuals are constantly suffering from negative moods, especially depression, that they are frequently hopeless, and that suicidal thinking and behavior is common. Persons who have BPD are often impulsive and reckless, have problems with irritability and hostility, and have great difficulty modulating their moods. You might be starting to realize now that there are many similarities between the features of the borderline diagnosis and the symptoms of mood disorders. In addition to their extremes of personality dimensions, persons who have borderline personality disorder frequently also appear to suffer from a mood disorder. In one study, 91 percent of patients being treated for borderline personality over a period of six years suffered at least one major depressive episode, and many experts have suggested a close connection between bipolar disorder and the borderline diagnosis.[6] We are making the point here that in thinking about persons with the borderline diagnosis, it is important to think about mood disorders as well. That's complication number one.

Self-Destructive Behaviors

A recent study of persons with a borderline diagnosis found that over 60 percent of them reported multiple suicide attempts, and about 70 percent reported multiple episodes of other kinds of non-life-threatening self-harm such as repeatedly cutting or burning themselves.[7] A similar study found that more than half of patients with the borderline diagnosis have an alcohol or drug problem.[8] Another study found that about half of these patients have some kind of problem with eating behaviors,[9] either the pattern of self-starvation and drastic weight loss called anorexia nervosa or the pattern of binging on huge amounts of food in a short period and then purging themselves of this food in some way (usually by making themselves vomit) called bulimia.

This is another set of problems that doesn't really seem to have much to do with personality traits (complication number two). You can see how some of the personality traits seen in persons with a borderline diagnosis can make these individuals more likely to engage in these behaviors—an impulsive person will be more likely to try cocaine when it is offered before thinking through the risks and consequences of doing so, or will be more likely to take an overdose during a moment of hopelessness, for example. Also, it's easy to see how persons with a poor ability to soothe themselves will be more likely to depend on alcohol and drugs to attempt to deal with their feelings. But these self-destructive behaviors are just that: *behaviors*. A simplistic but not unreasonable way to think about them is as very bad habits that persons who have BPD gradually develop and that become second-nature coping mechanisms after a while. They are another example of how the constellation of borderline features includes problems that are more than personality.

Traumatic Experiences

From the time that psychologists and psychiatrists first started to think about this group of patients and their problems, it became apparent that many persons who share the features of the borderline diagnosis have traumatic experiences of various types in their life story. Several studies have shown that persons with the borderline diagnosis are more likely than persons with other psychiatric diagnoses to report that they were victims of emotional, physical, or sexual abuse or neglect as children. Some research has focused on more subtle childhood difficulties such as death of a parent at an early age or absence of a parent for long periods, such as from a serious illness that necessitated a prolonged hospitalization. Early researchers also focused on a kind of emotional absence that they theorized takes place when a couple in a conflict-ridden, tumultuous marriage are so caught up in their own problems that their child doesn't get as much emotional nurturing as she otherwise would.

Not all persons with the borderline diagnosis have a history of abuse, and only a minority of persons who have had traumatic early life events develop severe mental health problems. Although an abuse history is clearly neither necessary nor sufficient to cause these problems, this connection has been replicated in too many studies to think of it as only a coincidence. The meaning of this connection is not at all clear; however, persons with an abuse history are known to have various psychological symptoms more often than those who do not, symptoms such as anxiety and depression, and they benefit from psychological treatments that help them put their traumatic past behind them.

Perhaps a traumatic history acts together with other factors, such as particular personality traits or risk genes for a mood disorder, to trigger the constellation of problems we are discussing in some individuals (complication number three). Paying attention to the possibility of a history of abuse, and addressing this issue at the appropriate time, is a necessary part of well-rounded treatment of these patients. In a later section, we will discuss this and the need for awareness of each individual life story for effective treatment.

The Bigger Picture

In this chapter, we've talked about personality and the concept of a personality disorder, but we've also given you some information suggesting that *personality* problems may not explain all the various difficulties these people experience. We've mentioned the high rate of mood disorders in people who have BPD and the high rate at which these people develop unhealthy and self-destructive behaviors. We've also shared with you that many (though not all) persons with the borderline diagnosis have had difficult, even traumatic events in their lives, and that understanding how people react to those kinds of experiences is important in developing their plan of treatment. This explains why we chose the title of this chapter, to make the point that the person who has BPD not only has problems that can be understood as an aspect of personality, but usually has other kinds of problems as well. They have problems of "personality" and *more*.

Some behavioral scientists have tried in various ways to bypass this complexity, for example, by suggesting that persons who get a diagnosis of borderline personality disorder "really" just have a mild form of bipolar disorder. Or by saying that what looks like a mood disorder in these individuals isn't "really" major depression or bipolar disorder but rather an expression of poor coping skills because of their personality traits. Or that all persons with this diagnosis have been abused (even if they don't remember it) and that focusing on abuse issues is the only necessary treatment.

We think that these are academic and not helpful "chicken-and-egg" arguments that distract us from reaching a deeper and individualized understanding of these problems. Even more important, such simplistic thinking can lead practitioners to ignore what we know about treating all patients with mental health concerns: that most patients have a combination of different kinds of problems that each need to be approached in different ways, approaches that vary depending on the unique combination of difficulties—and strengths—that the patient has. "One size fits all" simply isn't an adequate approach in medicine and especially not in psychiatry.

In part 2 of this book, we will continue to "unpack" the borderline diagnosis and review the different kinds of causes that underlie the various problems these individuals have.

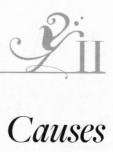

II

Causes

CHAPTER 3

The Four Faces of
Borderline Personality Disorder

Unlike other medical specialists, psychiatrists spend a lot of time arguing about how we should think about the problems we treat. Over many
decades, we've disagreed, for example, on whether alcoholism is better thought of as a reflection of personality weakness, or as a disease,
or perhaps as something else entirely. Throughout the 1960s and 1970s,
prominent psychiatric experts taught that the devastating mental illness schizophrenia was caused by *schizophrenogenic* (that is, schizophrenia causing) mothers who brought on their child's mental illness
through their rearing practices.[1] This particular idea has now been
completely discredited, and we know (or at least, *think* we know) that
schizophrenia is a biologically caused brain disease.

This disagreement illustrates why psychiatrists spend so much time
talking about how to conceptualize the problems we treat: with only a
few exceptions, we are very much in the dark about the basic causes of
psychiatric illness. This can make it difficult to know how best to treat
the difficulties that psychiatric patients face. We also know that mental health professionals not only treat mental illnesses but are called on
to help people who are distressed because of the natural feelings and
reactions they have when bad things happen to them. A person whose
spouse has recently died can benefit greatly from a few sessions with a
professional grief counselor, and no one would think that the sadness
and emptiness they feel for a time is a type of mental illness. Every individual has a unique combination of personal strengths and weaknesses
that help or hinder her in the ability to cope when bad things happen.
Obviously, it's important to think about all these different kinds of fac-

Table 3.1 The perspectives of psychiatry

The disease perspective considers:	what the patient *has*.
The dimensional perspective considers:	who the patient *is*.
The behavioral perspective considers:	what the patient *does*.
The life story perspective considers:	what the patient *encounters*.

tors when trying to decide how best to help an emotionally distressed person. Similarly, it's important to think about these factors when trying to comprehend the problems that persons with the borderline diagnosis face and in deciding how best to help them.

At Johns Hopkins, Drs. Paul McHugh and Phillip Slavney have spent several decades developing a logical and straightforward way of considering all these elements when trying to grasp the problems that psychiatric patients have and to make decisions about how to help them. We use their framework in this section to clarify borderline personality disorder and, in the next section, its treatment.

As we've already indicated, the problems that persons with the borderline diagnosis have often seem so complex as to be overwhelming. McHugh's and Slavney's framework, which they call the *perspectives* of psychiatry, helps tremendously in clarifying this complexity (see table 3.1).[2] More important, this approach guards against any oversimplification and the natural tendency to look for "one size fits all" treatment approaches. A word of warning: fully grasping this approach requires a step back from any current crisis, probably several re-readings of the paragraphs that follow, and a fair amount of thinking. You are about to take a mini-seminar in psychiatric thought. The effort will pay off, however, in a more complete and nuanced appreciation for the different kinds of problems these people face.

The Perspectives of Psychiatry

The first perspective is a familiar one: the medical, or *disease perspective*. Using this perspective, one considers *what the person has*. This is the way doctors think about their patients most of the time. They look for the disease, that is, the malfunctioning organ or body system, that explains the patient's symptoms.

A previously healthy young man comes to the emergency room with a high fever and painful, labored breathing. We know from centuries of medical experience that these are the symptoms of pneumonia, an infection of the lungs. And we know from the work of great medical pioneers like Louis Pasteur and Robert Koch that this patient's lungs are teeming with one of the several types of bacteria that cause pneumonia.

Another patient comes to the ER in an ambulance. She's a middle-aged woman with a history of high blood pressure who suddenly started to slur her words when speaking and now isn't able to move her right arm or leg. Again, medical experience tells the doctor that she has suffered what is commonly called a stroke and that a brain scan will show that blood is no longer flowing properly to a particular area of the left side of her brain.

In both of these patients, something has gone wrong with the body, a bacterial invader in one case, a blockage in a vital blood vessel brought on by years of elevated blood pressure in the other. A medical condition (or disease) has afflicted these previously healthy individuals.

In psychiatry, we now recognize that some conditions we treat are diseases too. We've already mentioned schizophrenia. Bipolar disorder and some forms of serious depression appear to be diseases as well. They occur in previously healthy individuals, and their symptoms are extremely similar from one patient to another. Brain changes have been demonstrated in these conditions, and they run in families—another indicator of something biological going on. Most compelling is that various chemical manipulations, namely the use of medications, can bring about symptom relief. In the case of mood disorders (bipolar disorder and serious depression), medication treatment can often take away the symptoms entirely and completely restore the individual to his previous level of health.

The second perspective of psychiatry provides a vantage point from which to consider *who the person is*. We discussed *personality* at length in chapter 2, and thinking about personality traits takes this perspective. As we emphasized in that chapter, people vary quite a bit in how prominent and dominating a particular personality trait is in them; thus McHugh and Slavney call this the *dimensional perspective,* to emphasize this variability on a continuum. To remind you of what is meant by personality, we'll again quote the great psychiatrist-turned-philosopher Karl Jaspers: "We see personality in the particular way an individual expresses himself, in the way he moves, how he experiences and reacts to situations, how he loves, grows jealous, how he conducts his life in general, what needs he has, what are his longings and aims, what are his ideals and how he shapes them, what values guide him and what he does, what he creates and how he acts."[3]

Psychologists have generally found that the best way to think about personality is as a collection of personal traits that vary in prominence from person to person. Some of us are natural risk takers, but some of us are risk averse. Some of us are gregarious and outgoing, and some are quieter and more serious. We all fall somewhere along these personality dimensions, and knowing where a particular person falls can be helpful in understanding her and knowing how best to help her with emotional problems. An important part of psychotherapy is helping individuals know themselves and their personality traits better so they can appreciate their strengths and weaknesses and grow. For example, someone who is having trouble maintaining relationships may discover during the course of therapy that she is extremely risk averse and gets uncomfortable in a relationship so quickly that it never has a chance to really develop. Helping a person recognize this about herself can help her see what is going on and develop strategies to work around personality vulnerabilities in order to solve problems.

This is a good point at which to pause for a moment and point out something important about the perspective method of thinking about psychiatric problems: the four psychiatric perspectives don't inform each other. That may sound odd and difficult to grasp, but some examples that focus on more familiar medical problems rather than psychiatric illness will make it clear.

Consider for a moment the first emergency room patient we presented to you earlier, the young man with pneumonia. When the doctor orders the hospital's clinical laboratory to examine a sample of the phlegm that the young man is coughing up, she doesn't expect to get any information about what kind of person he is. In other words, her reasoning about what is wrong with him from the *disease perspective* doesn't give her any information about how the *dimensional perspective* may be influencing his problem. In fact, reasoning from the dimensional perspective isn't at all helpful: thinking about whether he's a careless or precise fellow in his personal style, whether he's more or less outgoing, more or less sensitive to the needs of others, is a waste of time in this context. These issues explain nothing about what kind of bacteria is causing his pneumonia. Thus, information gained from the one perspective doesn't tell you anything about the other.

However, information gained from these different perspectives can have a powerful *additive* effect when it comes to developing treatment approaches for real people, and thinking about the patient in these different ways is usually important. Let's consider, for example, our other ER patient, the woman who is having a stroke. The doctor recognizes the symptoms of her stroke quickly and will order a brain scan to confirm the diagnosis and then prescribe blood clot–dissolving medication to minimize damage. However, the doctor also has some other important information about this patient: she has high blood pressure, a condition that puts her at much higher risk for a stroke. Imagine as well that the doctor finds out from the patient's husband that his wife isn't consistent in taking her blood pressure medication because she's a rather disorganized person who tends not to pay close attention to details. Let's imagine too that the patient's family doctor had prescribed two different blood pressure medications for this patient to take, including one that needs to be taken three times a day. The family doctor either didn't know about, or didn't pay attention to, *who this person is* (a bit disorganized and with poor attention to details) when he prescribed such a complicated regimen of blood pressure medication—to the patient's serious detriment. This patient, because of *who she is*, will have a difficult time keeping up with a complicated schedule of blood pressure medications.

Fortunately, there are blood pressure medications that can be taken only once a day, and several preparations combine two medications in just one tablet. What if, armed with better knowledge about the patient's personality traits, her family doctor had managed to devise a treatment plan for blood pressure control that involved taking just one pill once a day? Clearly, it would have been easier for this particular patient to keep up with this plan and thus more likely that her blood pressure would have been better controlled. Perhaps the stroke could have been prevented. Knowing about this patient's personality issues doesn't help much to make the diagnosis of high blood pressure and stroke, and knowing that she is having a stroke because of poorly controlled high blood pressure doesn't tell you anything about the strengths and weaknesses of her personality—the different perspectives don't inform each other. However, knowing not only *what the person has* but also *who the person is,* that is, using information gained from both these perspectives in thinking about this patient's treatment, will clearly result in a better long-term outcome for her.

The third perspective looks at *what the person does* and considers patterns of *behavior.* Psychological research has told us that if a particular action leads to the attainment of some desirable goal, all animals, including humans, will tend to repeat that behavior. Eating food gets rid of that uncomfortable empty feeling that we call "hunger," so we learn, early on, to eat when we are hungry. Drinking alcoholic beverages results in a pleasant, warm, sociable feeling that people enjoy and that causes them to want to continue drinking. They soon learn, however, that drinking too much will inevitably result in physical discomfort in the form of a hangover the next morning. So they learn to balance one goal against the other: they enjoy drinking for the pleasant feelings they get, but drink only in moderation to avoid the unpleasant consequences.

Culture and social forces also have a powerful effect on shaping behavior. For example, in Japan, a culture of heavy drinking by businessmen developed starting in the 1960s, when drinking to the point of extreme intoxication became an expected part of entertaining business clients and celebrating company successes.[4] In this case, being socially accepted became another motivation for alcohol use, despite the repercussions of excessive intoxication (psychologists refer to this as something that *reinforces* the behavior).

A behavior becomes problematic when the individual continues to do something that makes him feel good in some way despite worsening negative consequences that start taking a toll on his health and relationships. Sometimes, the negative effects can also have the perverse effect of further reinforcing the problem behavior. Problem drinking is a good example: some people drink to relieve uncomfortable feelings like depression or anxiety, but with repeated bouts of heavy drinking, once the immediate effects of the alcohol wear off, depression and anxiety are usually worse than they were at the beginning. Eventually, the person needs to use more and more alcohol to gain any temporary relief, sometimes to the point where alcohol doesn't make him feel good anymore, but just a little less bad and closer to normal—at this point, the individual is truly addicted to the behavior. Note that depression and anxiety didn't *cause* this person's problem behavior; they may have triggered it and have a role in sustaining it, but this habit has essentially taken on a life of its own as a way of dealing with uncomfortable feelings.

Substance abuse is the most common form of problematic behavior, and persons who have borderline personality disorder often suffer from addiction. They commonly have other behavior problems as well: cutting and self-mutilating behaviors, eating disorders, and repeated suicidal threats and actions. In all these cases, the individual engages in self-damaging behaviors that are motivated by some good feeling they bring on or some unpleasant feeling they help relieve. Individuals who cut on themselves frequently say they do so "to keep from feeling numb" or "to get the bad feelings from the inside to the outside." The self-starvation of the anorexic often starts out as a behavior that makes the individual feel more attractive and more in control of her body. Repeated overdoses may be desperate attempts to "block everything out" or "just go to sleep for a long time."

Treating problem behaviors consists of, perhaps most important, helping the person to see the behavior as a problem, and then to identify the goal or goals that the behavior accomplishes for him and to develop other ways of reaching that goal. One treatment approach for addiction asks the patient to make a list of the bad things about his addiction, but also the *good* things. It doesn't take people long to realize that there are many good things about addiction: the pleasurable feelings of being high, of course, but many other aspects as well. There is often the adventure and thrill of purchasing a drug like cocaine without getting arrested and the sense of independence and self-importance that comes from being a law-breaking rebel who flouts social conventions and expectations. There is the instant social acceptance and ready-made community of other addicted persons (remember the alcoholic Japanese businessmen?).

This technique recognizes that only when the person concludes that the negative consequences of the behavior outweigh the positive will he be willing to work on changing the behavior. This can be quite difficult. The person with cutting behaviors quickly learns that this behavior terrifies and intimidates those around him and gives him a power to manipulate others that can be difficult to give up. Often, people are not consciously aware of these advantages. Thus, helping them become aware is another important aspect of eliminating the behavior.

Other psychiatric perspectives play a role in understanding problem behaviors, even if they don't entirely explain them. Take, for example, one form of disordered eating behavior, anorexia nervosa. These individuals often suffer from mood disorders such as serious depression, illnesses that fill them with bad feelings about themselves that they don't know how to cope with. These negative self-attitudes may include thinking "I'm fat and ugly," and so the person starts dieting. If she is a self-disciplined individual who tends to be goal oriented, she will likely be successful at losing weight and feel a bit better about herself when friends and family compliment her on her new slimmer figure. This has the effect of reinforcing the dieting behavior, and she continues to diet to the point where constant hunger and poor nutrition start distorting her perception of her body and she loses control of the behavior, which then becomes self-sustaining and takes on a life of its own. In this case, *what the person has*—depression—interacts with *who the person is*—a self-disciplined and goal-oriented person—to trigger and help sustain *what the person does*—engage in abnormal eating behaviors.

The fourth perspective considers how *what the person has encoun-*

tered in his life may explain something about his distress. Examining the unique set of experiences that an individual has had during his lifetime and is encountering at present can reveal a lot about what will help him feel better. Getting patients to share their life story is a vital part of understanding this aspect of their difficulties and gives this last psychiatric perspective its name: the *life story perspective*. Think for a moment about the person who had the eating disorder described earlier. Imagine that this person tells her therapist that her mother had pressured her from a young age to enter beauty pageants for children, strictly controlling her diet and focusing attention on her appearance rather than on her other attributes or accomplishments. It's easy to see how this young woman might tend to be more focused on her appearance than other girls her age, thus essentially preparing the way for the development of an eating disorder. If this young woman's self-esteem is so tied to her appearance that she has difficulty valuing her other attributes, doing something to improve her appearance will be high on the list of things to do to feel better. This person's life story, *what she has encountered*, is an important part of the totality of her troubles. Therapy will help her begin to see and, more important, to appreciate the other aspects of herself that are good and valuable and to pay less attention to her appearance. But only listening to and appreciating her life story will reveal how important a part of her treatment this strategy will be.

Many clinical research studies have shown that many (though not all) of the persons who receive a BPD diagnosis have a history of abuse, often sexual abuse. We also know that people with abuse histories, especially sexual abuse, often have a damaged sense of identity and that a fairly specialized psychotherapeutic approach is necessary to repair their damaged identity, to help them make peace with their history and put it behind them so they can move on with their lives. Clearly, paying attention to *what the person has encountered* is vitally important in knowing how to help someone who has BPD.

PSYCHIATRY HAS GOTTEN INTO TROUBLE at various times over the past one hundred years or so by paying too much attention to those who preached that only one of these perspectives was sufficient to explain any and all of a patient's emotional or behavioral problems.

In the early twentieth century, the theory of *degeneration* attempted to do just this, proposing that inborn and inherited biological defects explained every form of mental illness, behavioral or social problem, and even personality quirks. As one modern psychologist put it, according to the theory of degeneration, "A host of individual and social pathologies . . . could be explained by a biologically based affliction . . . a wide range of social and medical deviations, including crime, violence, religious fanaticism, mysticism, insanity, absence of shame, impulsiveness, masturbation, vagrancy, alcoholism, prostitution, suicide, inertia, apathy, egotism, gambling, tattooing and pornography, could be explained by reference to a biological defect within the individual."[5] This might sound simply comical until one learns that this thinking, combined with the newly emerging field of genetics at the time, led to the development of *eugenics,* which purported to save mankind from these ills essentially through selective breeding. This thinking led to the sterilization of mentally retarded individuals in the United States and other countries and the murder of "mental defectives" by the Nazis. The disease perspective had run amuck.

The theory that certain parenting styles could cause schizophrenia, which had great sway in American psychiatry in the 1960s and 1970s, was the life story perspective run amuck.

The behavioral perspective had its day as well. In the 1950s, behavioral psychologists like B. F. Skinner proposed what they called "radical behaviorism," suggesting that all aspects of mental function—and dysfunction—were essentially behaviors that could be shaped and manipulated and that all forms of mental illness could be cured with the right type of behavioral reinforcement.

In each of these cases, and there are others as well, a theory arose that considered mental functioning and psychiatric problems from only one perspective. In every case, the theory was ultimately proved wrong, and often patients were harmed.

If this all seems too theoretical and pedantic, consider this: the diagnosis that we are considering in this book is called borderline *personal-*

ity disorder. This implies that all the problems of someone who has BPD can be understood as aspects of personality—it's just *who they are.* With only a moment's reflection (and assuming you read chapters 1 and 2), you can see that this is simply not the case.

CHAPTER 4

What the Person Has

The Disease Perspective

In this chapter, we consider those aspects of borderline personality disorder that seem best explained by some biological factor, or more precisely, by some aspect of biological functioning that appears not to be working correctly in these individuals. Just as the symptoms of childhood-onset diabetes can be explained by the body not producing the essential hormone insulin, some aspects of borderline personality appear to be best explained by problems in functioning in certain areas of the brain. The most important reason to understand what these aspects are is that a biological problem is usually most effectively helped by a biological intervention, which in the field of medicine usually means a medication.

Mood Disorders

Perhaps the most common psychiatric illness in persons with the diagnosis of borderline personality disorder is a *mood disorder* of one kind or another. You will remember that one of the most basic features of borderline personality disorder is difficulty with emotional modulation. Mood disorders are just such problems. The severe depressive illness that is often called clinical depression or, using one of the DSM terms, *major depressive disorder* is one of these. Another is the more complex and usually more difficult to diagnose illness that is now called *bipolar disorder* (formerly manic-depressive illness).

These illnesses appear to be caused by functional problems in the areas of the brain that are important for normal mood regulation. One requirement for normal functioning in the most important of these brain areas, the hippocampus, is its ability to constantly reinvigorate through the development of new brain cells (neurons) from stem cells in the brain as well as through the dynamic process of remodeling the connections between its different nerve cells. This capacity for remodeling is called *neuroplasticity*. (One of the meanings of the word *plastic* is "easily shaped or molded.") You can think of neuroplasticity as the neurons' responsiveness and ability to react to change and stress; it appears to be involved in memory and learning as well. (The symptoms of mood disorder include thinking and concentration problems in addition to mood changes.) Neuroplasticity may be a necessary part of maintaining mood within a normal range, somehow "tuning" the responsiveness of our mood state to experiences and environment.

Neuroscientists have demonstrated that effective medications in treating mood disorders enhance neuroplasticity in one way or another. Antidepressants appear to do so primarily by triggering the development of new nerve cells, and medications usually called *mood stabilizers* appear to do so through protective mechanisms, that is, shielding neurons from chemical stresses in the brain, perhaps prolonging their functional life and enhancing their ability to remodel.

Major Depressive Disorder

This form of severe depression most commonly occurs in episodes (called *major depressive episodes*) that, untreated, typically last about a year. They can, however, be briefer or much longer. Most persons with this illness have recurrent bouts of severe depression and long periods of being depression-free in between.

A smaller group of people with major depression develop a longer-term illness with depressive symptoms that wax and wane over many years but never go away entirely or for long. Sometimes these individuals are almost free of depression; other times, their depression can be incapacitating, but they struggle nearly all the time with some level of low mood and other depressive symptoms.

The good news for these individuals is that essentially all persons with major depression appear to benefit from medical treatment for their illness. This makes it vitally important that the diagnosis of major depression never get missed and that beneficial treatment with anti-depressant medication be extended as soon as possible.

The Symptoms of Major Depression

The two core symptoms of major depression that are usually present in persons experiencing it are (1) *depressed mood* and (2) a loss of one's ability to derive enjoyment and pleasure from anything, an experience that psychiatrists call *anhedonia*, from the Greek *an-* (without) and *hedone* (pleasure). This emotional state can be so severe that the person cannot experience any positive emotions at all and may feel as if she's even lost her feelings of love for her spouse, children, and other family members and friends. (One of our patients always managed to treat her husband with kindness and caring regardless of how deep her depression. It appeared that this was a relatively preserved area despite how low her mood became; however, when asked about it, she said that she *remembered* that she loved her husband, but could not *feel* love for him right now—she was essentially acting on remembered feelings.) At the least, those with anhedonia will lose interest in *doing* much of anything, even things they could usually count on enjoying.

Persons in a major depressive episode will also find that many of the normal functions of their body are disrupted. Sleep problems are the most common and most distressing of these difficulties; individuals may have terrible insomnia, or sometimes sleep too much. Whether they sleep too little or too much, however, they never feel rested and are troubled by fatigue and lack of energy. Appetite changes occur as well—either up or down—and this change is usually severe enough to cause a significant change in body weight. Many depressed persons suffer from other physical problems as well: constipation is common, as is a heavy feeling in the chest and other bodily discomforts. If the individuals already suffer from some painful condition, such as arthritis or back trouble, their pain will become more distressing and unbearable to them.

Table 4.1 Symptoms of major depression

Mood symptoms
    Depressed mood
    Dysphoric mood
    Pervasive constricted quality of mood
    Loss of ability to experience pleasure (anhedonia)
    Guilty feelings
    Loss of interest in usual activities
    Social withdrawal
    Suicidal thoughts

Cognitive (thinking) symptoms
    Poor concentration
    Poor memory
    Indecision
    Slowed thinking
    Loss of motivation

Bodily symptoms
    Sleep disturbance
        Insomnia
        Hypersomnia
    Appetite disturbance
        Weight loss
        Weight gain
    Fatigue
    Headaches
    Constipation
    Worsening of painful conditions

What might be called the thinking aspects of normal mental functioning, what are generally called *cognitive functions*, are also disrupted in persons with major depression. These include one's ability to concentrate and focus and to think a problem through to a solution, as well as memory functions. Because of these problems, studying or reading a book or newspaper is difficult; sometimes even following a show on television becomes impossible. One of our depressed patients, a successful student at Harvard, could focus on nothing more difficult than children's books for some time while recovering from depression. The symptoms of major depression are listed in table 4.1.

An important aspect of major depression that is not captured by a simple list of symptoms is that these symptoms go on all day, every day, unvaryingly, week after week, often month after month. This abnormal mood state is often described as *pervasive* (though not meant in the same way as it is used to describe personality, that is, unwavering over *decades*) and is unvarying. The mood is said to become *constricted*, and the normal ups and downs—the normal *reactiveness* of mood to external events—flatten out. The depressed person can't do anything to cheer himself up, so one cloud-covered hour just blends into the next.

Given the unrelenting misery of major depression, it may not be surprising that suicidal thinking is a common symptom as well. Because suicidal thoughts and attempts are especially common in borderline personality disorder and often entwined with other types of problems, we're going to put off a discussion of them to a later section. Briefly, suicidal thinking troubles many persons who have major depression, and some do make suicide attempts. Other individuals, however, seem to more easily reject thoughts of actually ending their life but nevertheless find that they have grown weary of living and wish that something would happen to end it, or that they could "go to sleep and just not wake up." The term *passive death wish* has been coined to describe these feelings.

The mood state of major depression is not simply an exaggeration of ordinary sadness. In fact, the feelings often have an alien, anguished quality that even the greatest writers have not felt capable of accurately describing. The Pulitzer Prize–winning author of the novel *Sophie's Choice*, the late William Styron, suffered from severe episodes of major depression later in life. Even he felt he could not accurately capture the feeling state that it inflicted on him. "If the pain were readily describable, most of the countless sufferers from this ancient affliction would have been able to confidently depict . . . their torment. Healthy people [cannot] imagine a form of torment so alien to everyday experience. For myself, the pain is most closely connected to drowning or suffocation—but even these images are off the mark."[1]

Another factor differentiating ordinary sadness from major depression is that normal feelings are always connected to events in our lives in some way. People become sad when they experience loss. This may be a literal loss, like the death of a loved one or the breakup of a relationship, or may be a more intangible but still meaningful loss, like the feelings of disappointment one would have at not getting accepted into one's first choice of college. People recover from these periods of bad feelings, often in only a few days, depending on the triggering event. Although the profound sadness of grief after the death of someone close to us can last much longer, even bereavement has a normal and quite predictable time course. This sadness too gradually fades as the survivor reconnects with other people and generally starts to resume other aspects of life. Sometimes, a major depressive episode follows and seems to have been precipitated by a life event. But even when this is the case, the severity of the symptoms and the fact that the bad feelings continue for many weeks, usually for many months, identify them as symptoms of an illness.

These descriptions may imply that a severe major depressive episode can be unmistakable and relatively easy to diagnose. While this is quite true sometimes, often it is not. If the depression is chronic, that is, long term, and despite the person's emotional misery, she is somewhat functional in most areas, the diagnosis can be difficult to discern. In individuals who have BPD, who frequently have crises and disappointments that never seem to end because of their other problems, it's easy to miss the diagnosis of major depression by explaining it away as an understandable reaction to ongoing frustrations and disappointments in their lives.

Many clinical research studies have demonstrated that persons with a borderline diagnosis frequently also experience major depressive episodes. In one study, over 90 percent of persons who had BPD either were having a major depressive episode as they entered the study or developed one during the six years of the study.[2]

Dysthymic Disorder

Some persons struggle with low mood and an inability to experience much joy or enthusiasm in their lives for years at a time. Although they don't experience symptoms with the disabling severity seen in major depression, these individuals don't differ that much in the *kinds* of depression symptoms they have. They may have chronic troubles with insomnia or a tendency to sleep too much, poor appetite or a tendency to overeat. They don't feel good about themselves, are pessimistic and sometimes even hopeless about their future, and have to push themselves to get things done. In the last several editions of the DSM, this kind of depressive illness has been called *dysthymic disorder*, from Greek roots that roughly translate as "bad spirits." It has been proposed to call this problem *chronic depressive disorder* in the next edition of the DSM and to recognize that many of these individuals go on to experience bouts of disabling depression, that is, major depressive episodes.

This type of depression tends to start earlier in life (sometimes even in childhood) and to run more strongly in families (indicating that it has a strong genetic component).

Bipolar Disorders

Some people who go through bouts of severe depression experience other types of abnormal mood as well. Some experience bouts of *elevated* mood, the opposite of depression, and some go through periods of severe irritability accompanied by agitation. In either case, there is a dramatic increase in energy level in addition to the mood change. Initially this "speedy" feeling is often pleasant, but before long, the agreeable energized feeling gives way to an uncomfortable restlessness. Similarly, their thought processes commonly feel sped up, and although they initially feel that they are thinking more clearly than normal, their thought soon becomes jumbled and disorganized. Their speech also speeds up and eventually becomes increasingly disorganized, and they jump from one idea to the next so quickly that they become impossible to understand.

As their mood becomes increasingly elevated, they start to feel overconfident and engage in reckless behaviors. These can range from driving too fast or spending too much money to completely losing inhibitions and engaging in promiscuous sexuality, traveling to dangerous neighborhoods to buy illegal drugs, or other self-endangering behaviors. The irritability may be so severe that the person becomes assaultive and dangerous.

These kinds of symptoms constitute what psychiatrists call *mania*, from a Greek word meaning "madness," and like full-blown major depression, severe mania is a clinical condition that is unmistakable, and a person in its throes is unmistakably ill.

But also like major depression, manic-type symptoms may be much milder in many people. Some individuals who have bipolar disorder have no full-blown manic symptoms with disorganized or dangerous behavior but only the "speedy," pleasant feelings and mildly reckless behaviors, a condition call *hypomania*, that is, "sub-mania." These individuals, who have periods of severe depression and of hypomania, are given the DSM diagnosis of *bipolar II disorder*, as opposed to *bipolar I disorder*, which is reserved for patients who experience major depressions and episodes of full-blown mania.

The Dangers of Hypomania

It may seem counterintuitive, but hypomania can be far more destructive than mania. There are several reasons for this. The main reason is that hypomanic individuals don't seem to be feeling or behaving abnormally. They may come off as simply more lively, energetic, or enthusiastic. At worst, they may seem pushy, overconfident, or just plain rude and obnoxious—but they don't seem mentally ill. This means that they can do foolish, even risky things without other people realizing that their judgment is impaired or questioning their behavior. One of us had a patient who bought several luxury cars from several different auto dealers over a single weekend while in a hypomanic state, able to do so without raising any suspicion at the dealerships. A hypomanic person may withdraw huge sums of money from his accounts and make unwise investments or fly to some exotic location for a spur-of-the-moment getaway. Hypomanic persons may impulsively quit jobs or start extramarital love affairs. Often, only family and close friends, people who know the hypomanic person quite well, will be able to tell that there is something different about him and recognize that his behavior is uncharacteristic and worrying.

Another reason why hypomania can be so destructive is that the person in a hypomanic state is not in the least uncomfortable and usually refuses to even consider that he may be thinking and behaving abnormally. Unlike depression, hypomania is usually not experienced as an abnormal mood by the hypomanic person. This makes it almost impossible to get him into treatment. Since hypomania may last for many weeks, or even many months, like a raging tornado it can cut a wide swath of destruction through a person's life, wreaking havoc on relationships, finances, career plans, even physical health, such that the individual may emerge bereft and broke, perhaps with a criminal record, an addiction, or a venereal disease.

Mixed Mood States

Yet a third type of abnormal mood state that can occur in a person who has bipolar disorder is a poorly characterized and even more poorly understood combination of depressive and manic symptoms that psychiatrists, for want of a better term, label *mixed states*. A person in a mixed state *simultaneously* experiences depressed and manic symptoms. Usually, this is a combination of the emotional tone of depression and the physicality of mania. The person feels down and distraught, even hopeless, but is also sped up in thinking and imbued with a kind of destructive activation that one of our patients once called her "black energy." The person feels terrible but is simultaneously overenergized and pressurized. People in this intensely uncomfortable state describe feeling "like I'm jumping out of my skin" or "like I'm going to explode."

Mixed states are dangerous because the person has negative, depressing thought patterns together with excess energy, restlessness, and an inner sense of pressure and tension, putting her at high risk for hurting herself with suicidal behaviors. An individual in a mixed state will often be propelled into various other self-destructive behaviors that are not immediately life threatening. Persons in mixed states may cut or burn themselves. They often say that these desperate behaviors help them shift a terrible inner pain and tension to "the outside" and that the physical pain is somehow easier to deal with than the painful agitation of a mixed state. Since many people with the diagnosis of borderline personality have these same behavioral problems, though sometimes for other reasons, it is obviously crucial to determine whether one of these mood states is driving these behaviors so that these individuals can be properly treated.

Although the predominant negative emotion of the mixed state is often despair, another negative emotion, anger, is also quite typical. Once more, it's easy to see what a dangerous combination this can be: an individual literally seething with fury and at the same time reckless, disinhibited, and full of tension and energy. When a person with serious depression also "has a terrible temper" or suffers from "attacks of rage," it's a red flag for the diagnosis of a bipolar disorder rather than major depression.

Many psychiatry textbooks (and the DSM-IV) state that individuals with bipolar II disorder, that is, persons who have major depressive episodes and periods of hypomania but not full-blown mania, do not experience mixed states. Any psychiatrist who treats mood disorder patients can tell you, however, that this is simply not the case. Many patients with bipolar II disorder have "mini–mixed states" that may last only a few hours. The term *dysphoric hypomania* has also been applied to these mood states. As with other mood disorder symptoms, these short-lived mixed states can be missed if they're explained away as just "temper tantrums" rather than recognized for what they are.

Many people who have brief mixed states call them "anxiety attacks" or "panic attacks" and may thus be erroneously treated for an anxiety problem rather than a mood problem. This is especially likely because anxiety is so commonly a feature of pure depressive illnesses. With careful questioning and evaluation, however (and perhaps most important, being open to the possibility), it is usually possible to elicit the mood features in these individuals. In these abnormal agitated moods, depression and hopelessness rather than fearfulness are the emotions beneath the surface, and a kind of malignant energy, rather than the rush of adrenaline set off by fear, is the fuel that feeds this fiery emotional state.

Bipolar Spectrum Disorders

Over the past ten years or so, a new term has started to appear in experts' discussions of mood disorders: *bipolar spectrum*. In the 1950s, psychiatrists usually thought about bipolar disorder and major depressive disorder as two quite separate illnesses. In fact, the term *unipolar depression* was often used for what is now called major depressive disorder to emphasize this juxtaposition.

This strict dichotomy started to break down a bit in the 1970s, when experts began to talk about the differences between two forms of bipolar disorder, bipolar I disorder (characterized by major depressive episodes and episodes of mania) and bipolar II disorder (characterized by major depressions and episodes of hypomania only). Gradually, however, it has become apparent that many individuals who don't fit neatly into either of these groups definitely have a mood disorder with some

Table 4.2 Warning signs of bipolar spectrum disorders

Brief major depressive episodes (3–6 months)

Increased appetite during depressions

Increased sleep and low energy during depressions

Onset prior to age 25

History of postpartum depression

Family history of bipolar disorder

Antidepressant treatment effective at first but then "wearing off"

Antidepressant-induced agitation

Source: Adapted from S. N. Ghaemi et al., "The bipolar spectrum and the antidepressant view of the world," *Journal of Psychiatric Practice* 7, no. 5 (2001): 287–97, and B. Kim et al., "Bipolarity in depressive patients without histories of diagnosis of bipolar disorder and the use of the mood disorder questionnaire for detecting bipolarity," *Comprehensive Psychiatry* 49, no. 5 (2008): 469–75.

bipolar features. One bipolar disorder expert coined terms for several of these subtle variations and wrote definitions for bipolar III and IV, and even bipolar II$\frac{1}{2}$, III$\frac{1}{2}$, and V.[3] These terms haven't caught on with many other experts, mostly because there are just too many variations of symptom patterns in individuals to formally name and describe each one. Instead, the term *bipolar spectrum disorder* is now used to capture them all.

Most of these people have predominantly, sometimes almost entirely, depressive symptoms and only a few bipolar features to indicate that their illness is not simply major depression. Despite the subtlety of their symptom presentation, distinguishing these individuals from those with pure major depressive disorder is critical because antidepressants can sometimes make them worse rather than better, exacerbating the cycling of their mood symptoms, making them more frequent and intense. Some bipolar spectrum features are listed in table 4.2.

Borderline or Bipolar?

Right about now, you might be thinking, "That's it! There's no such thing as borderline personality disorder; it's all bipolar!" If this were true, of course, we wouldn't have needed to write this book. Nevertheless, we can say with confidence that individuals are sometimes misdiagnosed with borderline personality disorder who indeed have an undiagnosed bipolar disorder (usually bipolar II or a bipolar spectrum disorder) and that the symptoms and behaviors in them that had been called "borderline" disappear entirely with the correct medication approach. Also, many persons who have borderline personality disorder have a bipolar disorder that, when untreated, makes it nearly impossible for them to benefit from treatment specifically for their borderline symptoms and behaviors. But other patients with the borderline diagnosis don't seem to benefit from the medication treatments for bipolar disorder. What is the relationship between these two problems?

One of the most careful research studies to take a look at this complicated question was done by a group of psychiatrists at Harvard led by John Gunderson, who has studied the borderline diagnosis for many years and is one of the leading experts on the disorder.[4] In this study, 196 individuals who were carefully diagnosed by experts as having BPD were also carefully evaluated, at the beginning of the study and annually over a period of four years, for bipolar I or bipolar II disorder. In this study, almost one in five patients with a diagnosis of BPD either came into the study with bipolar disorder or developed it during the four years they were followed. While this may seem like a very high percentage, it's important to remember that more than 80 percent of these patients did *not* have or develop a diagnosis of bipolar I or II disorder. Also, the researchers evaluated patients with other personality diagnoses and found that nearly 8 percent, or about one in twelve, also had or developed bipolar disorder.

This study found that, as a group, the persons who had BPD and were treated for their bipolar disorder symptoms continued to have difficulties in functioning and continued to need intensive treatment; that is, the diagnosis and treatment of their bipolar disorder did not dramatically improve their overall clinical status, at least during the four years of the study. To quote the study authors, "The bipolar diagnosis encourages individuals and their families to have unrealistic expectations about what medications can do." They caution, "Omitting the borderline personality disorder diagnosis diverts therapeutic efforts away from psychosocial interventions that can often make a remarkable difference." We won't argue with that, but we also think that, for all its strengths, this study may underestimate the percentage of persons with a borderline diagnosis who can benefit from treatment for bipolar disorder. This is mostly because this study did not attempt to count the patients who developed symptoms of bipolar spectrum disorder, which may represent as many as half of all cases of bipolar disorder.[5]

Another way to look at this question is to see whether persons with a borderline diagnosis benefit from medications that we know help in bipolar disorder. When the issue is approached in this way, there is solid evidence from research studies that many people who receive the diagnosis of BPD do indeed benefit greatly from the medications known to be effective in bipolar disorder. In one of these studies, persons with the borderline diagnosis were given either lamotrigine, a mood-stabilizing medication known to be effective in bipolar disorder, or a placebo, for eight weeks.[6] This study was especially interesting in that it looked not at the effect of the medication on *mood*, but rather at its effect on *anger*. During each week of the study, the research subjects filled out a questionnaire that measured five aspects of anger: "State–Anger," which was their subjective state of anger at the time of measurement; "Trait–Anger," their readiness to react with anger; "Anger–In," their tendency to repress anger; "Anger–Out," their tendency to direct anger outward; and "Anger–Control," their ability to keep their anger under control. The results were thoroughly analyzed and tabulated, but two pictures are worth a thousand words (see figure 4.1).

Figure 4.1 shows the dramatic contrast between the group that took lamotrigine and the group that was on the placebo, with a significant decrease in the lamotrigine subjects' tendency to direct anger outwardly, which was reduced by about 30 percent, and their ability to control their anger, which improved by nearly 20 percent. If those numbers don't seem exciting at first, digging into the data a bit makes them much more impressive. Since lamotrigine is always started at a very low dose, the lamotrigine subjects were on a dosage that is known to be effective only for the last three weeks of the study. But we know that individuals who have mood disorders usually continue to improve for many weeks after treatment begins; it is often several months before the full effect of a medication is apparent. This would suggest that, if these subjects had been followed for a longer period, the benefits of the medication would have been even more impressive.

Studies similar to this one have demonstrated encouraging results for several other medications that are known to help in bipolar disorder. We'll discuss them in more detail in chapter 9.

Picturing Borderline Personality in the Brain

There have been tremendous advances in the development of tools to evaluate brain functioning in humans; perhaps the most astonishing have been in the field of *neuroimaging*, the new science of taking pic-

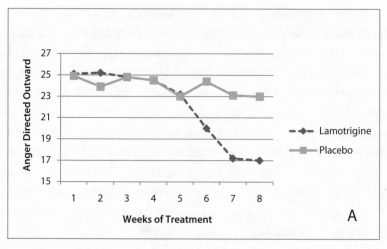

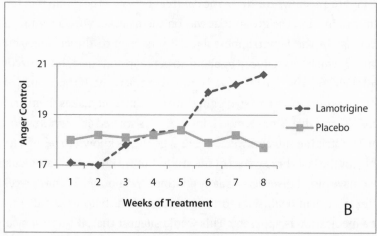

Figure 4.1. Improvement in anger management after eight weeks of treatment with lamotrigine. (A) Reduction of anger directed toward others on lamotrigine compared to placebo as indicated by the "Anger–Out" scale of the Trait Anger Expression Inventory; (B) increase of anger control on lamotrigine compared to placebo as indicated by the "Anger–Control" scale of the Trait Anger Expression Inventory. Modified from K. Tritt et al., "Lamotrigine treatment of aggression in female borderline patients: A randomized, double-blind, placebo-controlled study," *Journal of Psychopharmacology* 19, no. 3 (2005): 287–91.

tures of the brain. The scientists who use these techniques to study psychiatric illnesses are increasingly turning their attention to borderline personality disorder.

One of these techniques is *magnetic resonance imaging,* or MRI. This technology uses powerful magnets to "flip" water molecules in the brain in such a way that they emit particles that can be captured to form images. An MRI scan produces images of the body that are far more detailed than technologies that use x-rays, such as *computerized axial tomography,* or CAT scans. MRI scans of the brains of patients diagnosed with borderline personality syndrome compared with persons without the diagnosis demonstrate size differences in several brain centers. One of the most consistent findings is a reduction in the size of two brain areas known to be important in emotional regulation: the hippocampus and the amygdala.[7] These structures take their name from the Greek words for objects that early anatomists thought they resembled, the hippocampus from the word for "seahorse," and the amygdala from the word for "almond." The location of these centers deep within the brain is shown in figure 4.2.

One of the most striking of these studies showed a further relationship between self-injurious behaviors and the size of these brain structures in persons who have BPD: the more significant the self-injury history, the more significant the structural differences.[8]

Several more recently developed neuroimaging techniques do more than show detailed pictures of the brain. They allow researchers to observe the workings of the brain in living persons. One of these is essentially a variation on the MRI technique; by changing certain settings on an MRI machine, differences in blood flow in areas of the brain can be demonstrated. Measuring blood flow is another way of measuring how active a brain area is—more active areas require more oxygen and therefore greater blood flow. A subject being scanned can even be asked to perform some mental task during the scanning process, allowing the brain area that is called into action by the task to be identified by the change in blood flow. This type of scan, which allows researchers to literally see the brain in action, is known as a *functional* MRI (fMRI).

Researchers using fMRI and other functional scans have demon-

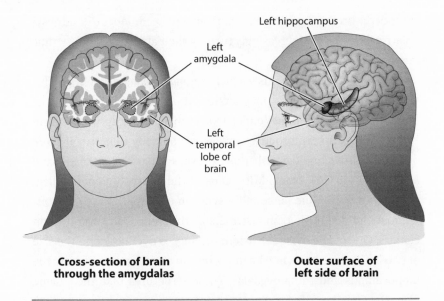

Left hippocampus

Left amygdala

Left temporal lobe of brain

Cross-section of brain through the amygdalas

Outer surface of left side of brain

Figure 4.2. The hippocampus and amygdala in the human brain. These structures play important roles in emotional modulation, mood, and memory.

strated decreased activity in other areas of the brain thought to be important for modulating strong emotions in persons who have BPD. Much of this work has focused on the amygdala and structures that it connects to. Previous research in both animals and humans has shown that this brain center is important in processing facial expressions in others, such as recognizing strong negative emotions like fear and anger in other people. The amygdala also appears to modulate the triggering of those same emotions in us. You can think of that "rush" of anger that you get when someone insults or mistreats you as your amygdala sounding off.

Using fMRI scanning, several groups of researchers have compared activity in the amygdala in subjects who have BPD to that in healthy control subjects as they were presented with photographs of people with various facial expressions.[9] They found that the individuals with a BPD diagnosis had much higher levels of activity in the amygdala than the healthy controls (figure 4.3). Even pictures of calm, neutral faces resulted in amygdala overactivity in persons who have this disorder.

These results have been interpreted to indicate that people who have BPD are likely to perceive negative emotions in others even when none are present. Remember, too, that one of the characteristics of persons who have borderline personality disorder is their tendency to become emotionally aroused quickly and have difficulties controlling emotions, especially negative emotions.

Another fMRI study flashed words on a screen in front of subjects

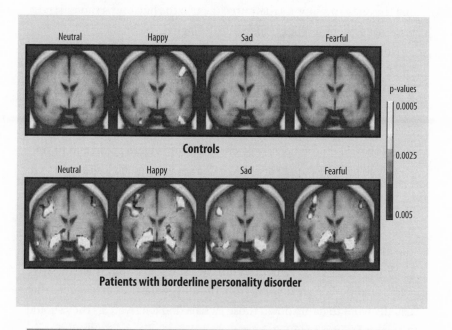

Figure 4.3. Composite functional MRI images from a neuroimaging study.
This study measured human brain activation triggered by looking at photographs of faces showing various emotions. The top row shows composite images of the control volunteers; the bottom row shows images from volunteers with a diagnosis of borderline personality disorder. The volunteers with the borderline diagnosis had a significantly greater increase of activity in their amygdalas, even when they were looking at neutral or happy faces. (The left side of figure 4.2 shows the location of the amygdalas viewed at this angle.) This was interpreted by the authors as indicating a tendency for even neutral human faces to trigger negative emotional reactions in persons with this diagnosis. Modified by Jacqueline Schaffer with permission from Elsevier, from Donegan et al., "Amygdala hyperreactivity in borderline personality disorder: Implications for emotional dysregulation," *Biol. Psychiatry* 54 (2003): 1284–93.

while they were actually in the MRI machine. Researchers asked the subjects to press a button if the word was printed in regular block letters, but not to press the button if the word appeared in *italics*. For example, if "FURNITURE" flashed on the screen, the subject would need to press the button, but if *"FURNITURE"* flashed on the screen (the same word in italics), they would need to suppress any urge to push the button. It turned out that several areas in the frontal cortex became more active in the subjects when one of the italicized words appeared and they had to suppress their urge to push the button, as though these brain areas were sending a "don't do it!" signal.

Here's where this experiment got really interesting: in addition to emotionally neutral words, like "furniture," the researchers also picked words that they reasoned would be especially charged for persons who have borderline personality disorder, such as "worthless" and "abandon" or positive words like "cheerful" and "tranquil." The researchers found that when the negatively charged words were presented to subjects who have BPD, the "don't do it!" areas were much less active than in the healthy controls. Also, the negative words caused greater activity in the amygdala of the BPD subjects than in the healthy controls. These researchers concluded that the study supported previous findings that the amygdala tends to be overactive in persons who have borderline personality disorder. This study also demonstrated that when negative emotional signals are coming from the amygdala, the cortex areas that usually work to damp down those signals don't activate as they should in someone who has BPD. Numerous other studies using similar techniques have found comparable alterations in brain functioning in persons who have borderline personality disorder.[10]

Despite these findings, these studies have not revealed the *causes* of the BPD aspects they investigated. Neuroimaging shows *what* is going on in the brain, but these studies do not answer *why* the brain is working this way in these individuals. The studies that show an overactive amygdala in these persons do not indicate *why* it is functioning that way. Is there some structural problem with the neurons in the amygdala? A difference in the way this center is wired? Or do these studies simply show the physical correlates of a purely psychological process?

Neuroimaging studies of depression demonstrate changes in blood flow to certain areas of the brain in depressed persons that disappear when the person recovers from depression—no matter what the treatment. BPD patients who receive dialectical behavioral therapy (DBT), a specific type of psychological treatment shown to be effective in helping with emotional dysregulation, show a reversal of the functional changes that characterize their condition, specifically, a reduction in amygdala overactivity.

These studies provide a window into the brain functioning of persons who have borderline personality disorder. They raise intriguing possibilities regarding potential new treatments, diagnostic methods, and perhaps ways to monitor the success of treatment. Unfortunately, these techniques are not yet refined enough to help assess treatment of particular individuals; all these studies have compared groups of patients with groups of healthy controls. But the day is not far off when technological improvements will allow these methods to become part and parcel of the way psychiatrists diagnose and monitor borderline personality disorder.

Genetics

Genetics is the study of heredity. Every high school student learns that each cell in the body of every living creature contains a set of instructions for its physical development and biological functioning, a marvelously simple code on a long spiral staircase of a molecule called DNA (deoxyribose nucleic acid). The transmission of DNA molecules, packaged into microscopic structures called chromosomes, from parents to offspring is the means by which we inherit the traits and qualities of our parents, from their eye color to their shoe size, their talents and their afflictions, the good, the bad, and the ugly—or the beautiful. (See www.dnai.org for an interactive introduction to the wonders of DNA.) If something goes awry in the process, some biological hiccup or another, or when the chance combination of otherwise trivial DNA variations adds up to a miscoded molecule in the offspring, disease can result. Sometimes one tiny change on one step of the DNA staircase can have catastrophic results, like sickle cell anemia or hemophilia, the "bleeding disease" that afflicted Queen Victoria's descendants. More often, many small anomalies combine with environmental factors to increase the risk of problems. Genetic risk is a substantial factor in the development of common illnesses like adult-onset diabetes, cancer, high blood pressure—and major depressive disorder, bipolar disorder, autism, and schizophrenia. Do genetic factors also contribute to the risk of developing borderline personality disorder? At present, the answer to that question is a qualified "maybe."

The first step in assessing the contribution of genetic factors to some condition is to assess whether it runs in families; this is a straightforward way of asking a somewhat more scientific-sounding question about some condition: do people who are more alike genetically tend to share the condition? An elegant way of approaching this question is to study twins. You may know that there are two different types of human twins: identical and fraternal. Identical twins develop when a fertilized ovum splits in half during its first cell division, and each cell separates and develops into a new fetus. Identical twins are genetic "clones"; each has exactly the same genes. Fraternal twins, on the other hand, develop when there happen to be two ova available for fertilization simultaneously and each develops into a fetus. Like ordinary siblings, fraternal twins share only half of their genes. Genetic studies of twins assess the rate at which twins either share a condition (they are said to be *concordant*) or do not share it (are *discordant*). If the assessment of many twin pairs demonstrates that identical twins are more frequently concordant for a condition than fraternal twins—that is, genetically similar individuals are more likely to share the condition—then genetics factors are shown to be a significant part of the risk for the condition.

This approach has been used to assess the borderline diagnosis and indicates that approximately half of the risk for the disorder is genetic.[11] One study showed a concordance rate of 35.3 percent among identical twins, meaning of identical twins with a BPD diagnosis, 35.3 percent of their co-twins were also diagnosed with BPD; the rate at which a fraternal twin's co-twin shared the diagnosis was 6.7 percent. Identical twins, sharing all their genes, were much more likely to also share the

BPD diagnosis than the fraternal twins. Another important point from this study is that genetics is only part of the story—about two-thirds of the identical twins' co-twins did *not* share their diagnosis, even though they shared *all* their genes. For the diagnosis of borderline personality disorder, like all other psychiatric diagnoses, genetics is not fate.

Advances in molecular genetics have resulted in the ability to check for hundreds of thousands of genetic markers in an individual for not much more than it costs to do a brain scan. This has made it possible to compare the pattern of genetic markers in a large group of persons who have a disorder to the pattern of markers in a group of healthy controls, looking for differences in the markers that identify particular genes. This type of project is called an *association study* because it attempts to discover whether particular markers are associated with the disorder. Association studies in borderline personality disorder have focused on a number of genes that are thought to be important for mood regulation and that have been linked to the size of the hippocampus. Several studies have indeed suggested that particular forms of these genes are associated with the diagnosis. One of these found an association between a particular form of a gene involved in the serotonin-signaling system in the brain (many antidepressant medications appear to enhance serotonin signaling) and the size of the amygdala in persons who have BPD,[12] thus linking to a finding from neuroimaging.

Like the neuroimaging studies, genetics research is beginning to shed light on the biological underpinnings of borderline personality disorder but is far from being clinically useful for individuals. It holds the promise, however, of leading to better diagnosis and treatment in the years to come.

CHAPTER 5

The Dimensions of Borderline Personality Disorder

In this chapter, we discuss how *who the person is* affects the symptom expression of borderline personality disorder and how this perspective informs its treatment. We hope that we made it clear in the last chapter why "personality disorder" is not really an accurate way to think about this disorder in its entirety. Nevertheless, everyone has a personality, and there are aspects of the BPD diagnosis that can best be understood from this perspective.

In our discussion of the meaning of personality and personality disorder in chapter 2, we presented the idea that personality is best understood as a collection of traits or qualities (things like loyalty, perseverance, dependability, inquisitiveness, risk taking, and so forth), and that every person's endowment of these traits can be discerned from an early age and remains relatively stable over time. We also presented the idea that a personality *disorder* exists when one or perhaps several of a person's personality traits are present to such an extreme that they consistently cause him to have trouble in relationships, social and occupational functioning, and other aspects of his life.

Measuring Personality Traits

One of the first persons to become interested in assessing and measuring personality was Sir Francis Galton (1822–1911). Galton was one of those extraordinary gentleman scientists of the nineteenth century who was interested in just about everything. He made significant contributions in scientific fields as diverse as statistics and meteorology.

He spent two years exploring Africa and was one of the first scientists to write about the implications of his distant cousin Charles Darwin's theory of evolution for human development. He coined the phrase "nature versus nurture" and expended many years of effort attempting to measure and quantify human traits, including personality traits.

Galton is credited with first proposing the *lexical hypothesis* of personality, which suggests that all the most important personality traits eventually find their way into our language, and further, that by analyzing language, it is possible to derive a comprehensive list of human personality traits. (*Lexical* is a term referring to words or vocabulary.)

In 1936, the American psychologists Gordon Allport and H. S. Odbert were curious to follow through with this idea of Galton's, and they went looking for all the personality-describing words in the English language. Using dictionaries to find nearly 18,000 candidates, they then distilled this list into a catalog of about 4,500 that they published in what they called a "Psycholexical Study."[1]

Several years later, another American psychologist, Raymond Cattell (1905–1998), decided to take things to the next logical step. He took the Allport-Odbert list of words and, by eliminating synonyms, reduced the number of personality-describing words in that catalog to 171. He then asked research participants to fill out questionnaires in which they used the words to rate people they knew on how well the words applied to them. Cattell then used a relatively new type of statistical technique called *factor analysis* to whittle the list down further. This technique can be thought of as another way of combining words that, for practical purposes, express the same quality. For example, the words "loyalty" and "dependability" aren't really synonyms, but when you think about real people, it's extremely likely that a person you would rate as highly loyal would also be quite dependable—and vice versa. In other words, measuring "loyalty" and "dependability" in a person is really measuring a single underlying *factor* that includes them both (hence the name of this type of analysis). Using this method, Cattell distilled his original list of 171 words to just 16 factors. (One of these, which he called "dutifulness," would seem to capture the two qualities in our example.)[2]

In the late 1950s, two U.S. Air Force researchers, Ernest Tupes and

Raymond Christal, asked 790 class members of the Air Force Officer Candidate School to rate each other on thirty-five of the personality factors identified in Cattell's work and reanalyzed similar datasets that had been published using other large samples, again using factor analysis.[3] Such a large number of subjects made for much more powerful results, and their factor analysis boiled the personality data down to just five factors (sometimes referred to as "the Big Five"), and to make a long story short, fifty more years of work by many other researchers have confirmed their results.

Questionnaires based on the five-factor model have now become the most widely used instruments for the assessment and study of personality. Several different questionnaires have been shown quite reliable in assessing the factors in individuals, questionnaires that a person can fill out in a short period (as little as 15 minutes for one of them). It is not necessary for a trained professional to administer these tests, and a computer can score them quickly. (As of this writing, you can take a five-factor-based test online and see your profile almost instantly.) The most widely used of these questionnaires is called the NEO-Five Factor Inventory (NEO-FFI), a sixty-item questionnaire that takes its name from three of the five factors (neuroticism, extroversion, and openness); it was developed by Paul Costa and Robert McCrae, both psychologists at the National Institute on Aging.

The Five-Factor Model of Personality

There are two important points to remember about the five-factor model when applying it to individuals who have psychiatric disorders: an important strength and an important weakness.

The strength is that the model was not developed based on a theory of psychology or personality development. The only assumption it makes is that the words we use to describe people really do describe *something* about them; that is, it is based primarily on the lexical hypothesis.* Most other personality models make assumptions about

*Another body of work that contributed to the development of the five factors *was* based on psychological questionnaires, which, in turn, were often based on a theory of

Table 5.1 The Big Five of five-factor theory of personality and their facets

Neuroticism	Conscientiousness
Anxiety	Sense of competence
Angry hostility	Orderliness
Moodiness/contentment	Sense of responsibility
Self-consciousness	Achievement striving
Self-indulgence	Self-discipline
Sensitivity to stress	Deliberateness
Extroversion	Agreeableness
Warmth	Trust in others
Gregariousness	Sincerity
Assertiveness	Altruism
Activity level	Compliance
Excitement-seeking	Modesty
Positive emotions	Sympathy
Openness	
Imagination	
Artistic interests	
Depth of emotions	
Willingness to experiment	
Intellectual curiosity	
Tolerance for diversity	

which personality factors or traits are "real," and then go about trying to measure them. The five-factor model makes no such assumptions.

The "weakness" of the model is that it was developed by research done on the general population, that is, on persons who, for the most part, did not have psychiatric problems. This means that using it to understand persons who have such problems needs to be done very cautiously.

So what are these five factors? Table 5.1 lists them, and table 5.2 provides short descriptions. Note that each factor comprises six subfactors, called *facets*, which can be thought of as aspects, or components, of each factor.

---

personality. This line of research, however, consistently replicated the factors found by Tupes and Christal, and the two approaches essentially merged in the 1970s.

Table 5.2 Descriptions of the Big Five personality factors

Neuroticism: The tendency to experience negative emotions, such as anger, anxiety, and depression

Those who score high in neuroticism tend to be:
- emotionally reactive and vulnerable to stress
- more likely to interpret ordinary situations as threatening and minor frustrations as hopelessly difficult
- have negative emotions that persist for longer periods

Persons who score low on neuroticism tend to be:
- less easily upset and less emotionally reactive
- calm, emotionally stable, and free from persistent negative feelings
  –Freedom from negative feelings does *not* mean that low scorers experience a lot of positive feelings.

Extroversion: The tendency to experience positive emotions, such as self-confidence, sociability, and assertiveness and to be engaged with the external world

Those who score high on extroversion tend to be:
- outgoing and talkative
- competitive and decisive
- adventurous and energetic
- drawn to social situations, where they are talkative, assertive, and draw attention to themselves

Persons who score low on extroversion tend to be:
- quiet, low key, and deliberate
- less involved in the social world
  –Their lack of social involvement should not be interpreted as shyness or depression; they simply need less stimulation and more time alone. They may be very active and energetic, though not socially.

Openness: The tendency to appreciate new and unusual ideas, to be interested in aesthetic and intellectual pursuits, and to seek out a greater variety of experiences

Those who score high on openness tend to be:
- intellectually curious, appreciative of art, and sensitive to beauty
- eager for new experiences
- more creative and aware of their feelings
- more likely to hold unconventional beliefs

People with low scores on openness tend to be:
- more conventional and traditional in their interests

- more comfortable with the plain, straightforward, and obvious rather than the complex, ambiguous, and subtle
  - They may find the arts and sciences uninteresting, or even view them with suspicion.

Conscientiousness: The tendency to be thorough, neat, well organized, diligent, and achievement oriented

Those who score high on conscientiousness tend to be:
- careful and deliberative, thinking before acting
- disciplined and acting according to the dictates of conscience
- hard working and reliable

People with low scores on conscientiousness tend to be:
- less goal oriented, less driven by success
- impulsive
  - They are not necessarily lazy or immoral, simply more laid back.

Agreeableness: The tendency to be compassionate and cooperative, to be concerned for social harmony, and to value getting along with others

People who score high on agreeableness tend to be:
- considerate, friendly, helpful, and willing to compromise their interests with others
- altruistic, nurturing, caring, and emotionally supportive of others
- optimistic about human nature, believing people are basically honest, decent, and trustworthy

Those who score low on agreeableness tend to be:
- unconcerned with others' well-being, and less likely to extend themselves for other people
- self-interested more than interested in getting along with others
- skeptical about others' motives
  - This can cause them to be unfriendly, uncooperative, suspicious, and even antagonistic toward others.

The five-factor model hypothesizes that these are the basic elements of personality present in every individual and that you can assess and describe the personality of individuals quite comprehensively by measuring these traits. In chapter 3, we said that one of the important perspectives needed to assess persons' psychiatric troubles is a *dimensional* approach, that is, thinking about how a person's personality traits compare to those of other people. The five-factor model takes exactly this approach; it assumes that these five basic personality elements are present to a degree in everyone and sets out to measure just where the person being tested compares to the general population's profile. The actual scores on tests such as the NEO-FFI are usually reported as percentiles, meaning that if a person scores an 80 on one of the scales, this means that 80 percent of the general population will score lower than this person and only 20 percent will have a higher score (the scores are corrected for gender, age, and other demographic factors).

Studies have been done to determine whether particular five-factor profiles are correlated with job satisfaction in trauma surgeons (the satisfied ones tend to be more extroverted),[4] what personality traits predict healthier dietary habits (more conscientious individuals eat a more healthful diet),[5] which traits indicate a risk for cigarette smoking (smokers score higher on neuroticism and lower on extroversion than the general population),[6] and the trait correlation for many other conditions and behaviors.

When analyzed using the five-factor model, the personality traits of people who have BPD have consistently scored high on the neuroticism scale and low on the extroversion scale. Several studies have also shown that persons who have BPD tend to test low on the conscientiousness and agreeableness scales.

Traits and "States"

Before we delve into these findings, it's important to talk in more detail about the weakness of the five-factor model—that it was developed by assessing individuals without psychiatric problems. It has, in fact, been demonstrated that the symptoms of psychiatric illnesses affect the results obtained on the five-factor testing. This is a problem for any kind of personality testing: current emotional *states*—symptoms like depression, anxiety, and so forth—show up in personality testing as if they were reflective of personality *traits*. For example, persons suffering from the symptoms of a major depressive episode score higher on the neuroticism and lower on the extroversion scales, but this finding has been demonstrated to disappear when the symptoms of depression get better after treatment with antidepressant medication.[7] Now obviously, someone's personality doesn't change over the few weeks it takes for his depressive illness to improve on medication, so it's important to somehow correct for this phenomenon when looking at the results of personality testing in the BPD diagnosis, that is, not to mistake what looks like a pattern of extreme personality traits on personality testing that is actually a distortion caused by emotional states.

A group of researchers headed by Dr. Mary Zanarini at the McLean Hospital in Boston studied several hundred persons with the BPD diagnosis over a period of ten years, a project that has yielded a treasure trove of data on the course of this disorder over time. (One of their findings, which we shall review in more detail in a later chapter, is that most patients with this diagnosis improve over time with treatment and that it should be thought of as a "good prognosis" psychiatric disorder.) As part of this study, they administered the NEO-FFI every other year to persons who had borderline personality disorder and who were receiving treatment for their problems. They found that, as a group, the persons' scores on the conscientiousness and agreeableness scales rose significantly over time—but the higher scores on neuroticism and lower scores on extroversion remained relatively unchanged.[8] These findings led them to propose what they term a "complex" model of the borderline diagnosis. As you will see, however, the model is really not that complex—not, that is, if you read chapter 3 of this book. They suggest that these persons can be thought of as having *acute symptoms,* which include mostly self-destructive behaviors, such as repeated suicide attempts and other self-harming behaviors, that often respond quickly to treatment, but also *temperamental symptoms,* which are for the most part a propensity to experience "chronic unpleasant emotions," such as anger, depression, anxiety, helplessness, loneliness, and impulsiveness, problems that change only slowly with treatment. We can express this same idea using McHugh's and Slavney's psychiatric perspectives by simply substituting "behavioral problems" for "acute symptoms" and "extremes of personality dimensions" for "temperamental symptoms."

The "Personality" in Borderline Personality

The most consistently replicated of the personality findings in border-line personality disorder with psychological testing based on the five-factor model is the high score on the neuroticism scale. While scores on this scale are elevated in people with just about any kind of psychiatric disorder, individuals with borderline personality disorder score not only much higher than healthy controls, but also substantially higher than people who have major depression or other types of personality disorders.

Before we go any further, a comment on the term *neuroticism* is in order. We can't say for sure why this factor continues to bear this anti-quated and pejorative name, and it is certainly an unfortunate choice for many reasons. It dates to a time when many psychiatric problems were called nervous disorders, and *neurosis* was used to refer to more severe psychiatric problems (such as bipolar disorder and schizophre-nia) that were not thought to represent a disease state. Neuroticism was the label chosen by the early personality researcher Hans Eysenck for a hypothesized personality trait that is largely the same as the five-factor model trait that shares its name. It is the only one of the five factors with a label that has a negative rather than a positive connotation (like agreeable and conscientious) and that clearly implies psychiatric disorder. The names for the five factors have been described as result-ing from "historical accidents, conceptual positions, and the entrench-ment that comes from a published body of literature,"[9] and perhaps that is the best explanation we can offer. It has been proposed to change the name of this scale to "emotionality" or even to its opposite, "emotional stability" (instead of high on "neuroticism," these same individuals would score low on "emotional stability"), or simply to label all factors by their first letter (making "neuroticism" simply "factor N"). But none of these ideas has caught on, so we're stuck with neuroticism and all its negativity.

How should we think of this factor in a real person? What would that person be like? Here's a description from Dr. Robert McCrae, one of the psychologists who developed the NEO-FFI (who, by the way, belongs to the "first initial only, please" camp): "N represents individual differences in the tendency to experience distress . . . High N scorers experience chronic negative [emotions]. The recurrent nervous tension, depression, frustration, guilt, and self-consciousness that such individuals feel is often associated with irrational thinking, low self-esteem, poor control of impulses and cravings, [bodily] complaints, and ineffective coping."[9]

In a 1984 paper, psychologists David Watson and Lee Anna Clark of Washington University wrote about this personality element in great detail. When the paper was written, the labels for the factors weren't quite settled, and they used the term *negative affectivity*, or simply NA (they criticized use of the term *neuroticism* as "slightly quaint"). The word *affect* can be thought of as referring to the personal experience of a feeling or emotion. "Negative affectivity . . . represents the extent to which a person feels upset or unpleasantly aroused versus peaceful. High negative affect includes a wide variety of unpleasant states (e.g., 'distressed,' 'nervous,' 'angry,' 'guilty,' and 'scornful'), whereas low negative affect is marked by terms such as 'calm' and 'relaxed' . . . It also includes such states as anger, scorn, revulsion, guilt, self-dissatisfaction, a sense of rejection, and, to some extent, sadness."[10]

They also emphasized that this propensity toward negative emotions is a pervasive feature of these individuals and doesn't simply mean that they react only with negative emotions when under stress. "Although an individual's mood will, of course, fluctuate widely, partly in response to specific situational factors, those high in NA will tend to report more negative affect across time and regardless of the situation. We are not arguing that high NA individuals report a consistently high level of negative affect. Rather, such individuals are, in any given situation, *more likely* to experience a significant level of distress."

In both papers, the authors caution that individuals with low neuroticism, who tend to be less troubled by negative emotions, are not necessarily full of positive emotions. Watson and Clark write, "NA is unrelated to an individual's experience of the positive emotions; that is, a high NA level does not necessarily imply a lack of joy, excitement, or enthusiasm." McCrae writes, "Individuals low in N are not necessarily high in positive mental health . . . they are simply calm, relaxed, even-tempered, unflappable."

These caveats highlight the fact that another of the five factors measures the capacity for positive emotions, namely *extroversion* (the term does not, as is usually thought, simply refer to sociability). Watson and Clark describe the positive connotations of this factor: "High positive affect is most clearly defined by words such as 'active,' 'excited,' 'alert,' 'enthusiastic,' and 'strong'—all very pleasant, positive emotions." McCrae clarifies, "The tendency to experience positive and negative emotions are not opposites . . . People who are cheerful, enthusiastic, optimistic, and energetic are not necessarily low in anxiety or depression—that depends on their level of N. But cheerful people consistently tend to be dominant, talkative, sociable, and warm." As you may remember, the other fairly consistent finding in individuals who have borderline personality disorder is that they tend to score low on the extroversion factor.

At this point, you may be thinking, "Wow, this is it! Borderline personality disorder really is a *personality* disorder." In the last chapter, after we described the symptoms and abnormal mood states of bipolar disorder, we cautioned you against jumping to the conclusion that everything about borderline personality disorder can be understood as simply the symptoms of bipolar disorder. Well, now we similarly warn you against concluding, "It's all personality."

Such a conclusion is certainly understandable. Our descriptions of symptom profiles in earlier chapters repeatedly emphasized that people with this diagnosis suffer nearly continuously from the whole gamut of negative feelings. Dr. Zanarini's list of "temperamental symptoms" (anger, depression, anxiety, helplessness, loneliness, impulsiveness) fits exactly into the profile of a person with a very high neuroticism score. We would agree that these extremes of personality are an important part of this disorder, perhaps even the most important factor to consider to make sense of it. But as we warned in the first section of this book, relying too much on just one perspective to comprehend as complicated a problem as borderline personality disorder is perilous. How does one decide whether pervasive feelings of depression, anxiety, and helplessness represent high neuroticism or are the symptoms of a mood disorder like major depression? At the risk of sounding flippant, we'll just say that it's really, really difficult—and that's why psychiatrists need so many years of medical training to do what we do.

Where Do Personality Traits Come From?

Imagine a newborn infant: helpless, completely dependent on others for everything, a creature totally lacking in any kind of knowledge or experience to guide its behavior, a creature whose biological endowment determines everything about it. Now think of an elderly person, worldly wise, with a lifetime of experiences—both good and bad—that inform her actions and behavioral choices. Intuitively, it make sense that our life experiences have an important role in shaping who we are, that is, our *personality*.

But you may remember that in psychologists Stella Chess and Alexander Thomas's studies of babies and children in the 1950s (discussed in chapter 2), aspects of personality can be discerned even in newborns. They found that it was possible to classify babies as "easy," "difficult," and "slow to warm up," even before they had any experiences at all, suggesting that biology must have at least some effect on temperament.

These two facts suggest that our personality must derive from some combination of our biological endowment, presumably largely determined genetically, and our life experiences (we'll leave out metaphysical considerations, such as divine intervention and planetary influences). Is it possible to separate these different factors and determine which is more important? Some geneticists have proposed that by studying twins, they can do just that.

First, a review of some facts about twins: remember that identical twins are exactly alike genetically, like clones; they share 100 percent of their genetic material. Fraternal twins, like brothers and sisters, share only 50 percent of their genetic material. This means that identical twins will *always* share a condition that is caused *completely* by genetic endowment, but that fraternal twins have only a 50 percent chance of both having the same condition. What about the environment and experience of twins? A lot of the environment that twins experience is the same, especially when they are young (factors like the parenting style of their parents and socioeconomic factors) and one would expect that *all* twins, whether fraternal or identical, will *always* share traits that are due entirely to their common environment. Let's think about "English as a native language" as a trait (it's not a personality trait, but a personal characteristic nonetheless). All twins, regardless of whether they are identical or fraternal, will always have the same native language (unless they were raised apart from birth, of course). This sharing of the characteristic is due to their common experience of growing up in an English-speaking family. But what if, as adults, one twin, but not the other, also spoke French? Not so difficult to imagine—perhaps one twin took French lessons and lived in Paris for a time and the other did not. In this case, "French-speaking" is a characteristic that is due to the one twin's *unique* experience, living in Paris. A pair of twins will *never* share characteristics that are due to each twin's *unique* environment.

So you can see that by examining the frequency with which twins share or do not share a particular characteristic, and carefully taking into account the pattern of differences in sharing rates between identical and fraternal twins, one can come up with the relative contributions of genetics, shared environment, and unique environments to that characteristic. (More sophisticated methods also attempt to quantify interactions between genetic endowment and the environment.)

In the 1990s, several psychologists (including NEO-FFI developers Paul Costa and Robert McCrae) asked over 800 pairs of identical and fraternal twins to rate themselves on questionnaires that measured the Big Five personality traits and analyzed the extent to which the twins matched on the Big Five. Using a sophisticated statistical method called *model fitting,* based on the sorts of assumptions about trait sharing between twins described in the section above, they calculated the relative contributions of genetics, shared environment, and unique environment to personality factors.[11] They found that genetic factors account for a little over half of an individual's differences in personality traits, with unique environmental factors accounting for the rest. Shared environment seemed to make essentially no contribution. The

authors concluded that "51 percent to 58 percent of individual difference variation along the Big Five dimensions is genetic in origin, 42
percent to 49 percent is due to experience unique to the individual, to
temporary situational factors, and to gene-environment interaction,
and none is due to effects of environment shared by the twins."

This last finding does seem odd, but the authors explain it by stating
that "whatever happens to individuals that makes a lasting difference is
mostly independent of their families . . . or has effects that are unique
to the individual."

So personality appears to be molded by our genes and our environment and experiences, as well as interactions between the two. This
perhaps rather unsatisfying result puts personality traits in good company with other complex human qualities such as intelligence, which
also appears to result similarly from varying contributions of nature
and nurture.

Conclusions about Personality and the Borderline Diagnosis

These findings about the origins of our personality, that personality is
determined in about equal parts by genes *and* environment, fit pretty
well with what we know from observing the personalities of real people over time. Common experience reveals that personality evolves in
response to life events, shifts in cultural values, and the lessons we learn
from simply living life. But the fact that personality has a significant
genetic component suggests that such change will be slow and incre-
mental. This is indeed what studies have shown. Repeatedly measuring
personality traits with the five-factor model over many years in individuals has shown that the usual pattern is a decrease in neuroticism
(that is, more emotional stability) and increases in conscientiousness
and agreeableness.[12] That sounds like a pretty good definition of matu-
rity, doesn't it? Studies have also shown that psychotherapy has similar
effects. In one study of persons with several different types of personality disorders, neuroticism decreased and agreeableness increased after
a year of psychotherapy.[13]

We can conclude that many of the problems that persons with the borderline diagnosis suffer from do indeed seem best understood as extremes of personality, specifically a deep-rooted tendency to experience negative and unpleasant emotions, which are provoked easily in them by any number of stresses, both extreme ones and trivial ones. Fortunately, this same aspect of personality, called "neuroticism" by personality researchers, decreases over time simply as a result of the natural maturing process. Even more fortunately, with psychological treatment, this improvement process can occur much more quickly.

CHAPTER 6

Behaviors I

Addiction and Eating Disorders

In this chapter and the next, we consider those aspects of borderline personality disorder that appear to be best explained as problems of behavior. Behaviors, quite simply, are *what we do*. The patterns or rules that characterize behavior were first examined over a hundred years ago by the famous Russian psychologist Ivan Pavlov (1849–1936), who was awarded the Nobel Prize for his accomplishments.

The basic principles of behavioral psychology are quite simple: when something we do makes us feel good, we are apt to continue doing it; when something we do makes us feel bad, we are apt to stop the behavior. Behavioral psychologists call the "feeling good" part of the process *positive reinforcement,* and its opposite, *negative reinforcement.* A child may touch a hot stove once or even twice, but the painful consequences of doing so (the negative reinforcement) prevent the child from engaging in this behavior more than a few times. Receiving praise or maybe a gold star for a good grade on a test (positive reinforcement) encourages a child to keep up the good work. The evolutionary advantage of these rules is obvious, and these patterns seem hard-wired in most animals; we use these principles to mold the behaviors of our pets, and the same principles can be demonstrated to operate in creatures as simple as fruit flies and pond snails.[1]

A behavior disorder develops when there is some imbalance between positive and negative reinforcement, such that the individual continues to engage in some particular behavior despite increasingly grave consequences.

Addictive behaviors are the easiest to understand in this way. An alcoholic drink gives most people a warm, relaxed feeling that is quite pleasant. But people quickly learn that overindulging has negative consequences—that foggy, miserable feeling we call a hangover. Most of the time, this negative reinforcement results in people learning to moderate their drinking behavior. Some individuals, however, continue to drink excessively despite increasingly grave negative consequences, like problems in their relationships and even serious health problems.

Often (but not always) there is some other factor that sustains the unhealthy behaviors; for example, individuals who have not developed healthy and effective psychological coping mechanisms may turn to alcohol or drugs as a way to cope with psychological stresses. Individuals who are overwhelmed by emotional pain do the same to anesthetize themselves from these feelings. It should be fairly clear to you now that persons who have borderline personality disorder experience both problems: inadequate coping mechanisms and an abundance of emotional pain. Using this model to understand other behavioral problems, such as eating disorders and self-harming behaviors, is not quite so intuitive. But we believe that with a little explanation, you will agree that the model makes a lot of sense in illuminating these problems as well.

In the rest of this chapter, we discuss addictions and eating disorders, behavioral problems that trouble many people who have the borderline diagnosis. We'll need a whole chapter to discuss self-harming behaviors, so we will spend the next one on self-mutilation and suicidal behavior.

Alcohol and Drug Addiction

About half of individuals with the diagnosis of borderline personality disorder also have some form of addiction to alcohol or illegal drugs.[2] The substances they abuse run the gamut from alcohol to marijuana to "hard drugs" like cocaine (table 6.1). A study that followed persons who have BPD over a period of seven years revealed that even those who did not have an addiction problem at the start of the study had a greater than one in ten chance of developing one during the course of the

Table 6.1 Substance use in 137 patients with borderline personality disorder

Substance abused	Number of patients	Percentage of patients	Percentage of total substances abused*
Alcohol	67	48.9	29.4
Tranquilizers	64	46.7	28.1
Cannabis	33	24.1	14.5
Cocaine	22	16.1	9.6
Narcotics (pain medications)	20	14.6	8.8
Stimulants ("uppers")	16	11.7	7.0
Hallucinogens	5	3.6	2.2
PCP	1	1.0	1.0

Source: Adapted from R. A. Dulit et al., "Substance use in borderline personality disorder," *American Journal of Psychiatry* 147, no. 8 (1990): 1002–7.
* Percentages add up to greater than 100% because some patients abused more than one substance.

study.[3] This was true even if other symptoms improved. These results have been interpreted as indicating that those who have BPD may remain at risk for substance abuse problems throughout their lives and need to be vigilant against using alcohol or drugs to cope with bad feelings over the long term. Substance use as a coping strategy can quickly trap them in an addiction, with all its associated risks and problems.

Alcoholism

Alcoholism is the most common substance abuse problem in the United States. Since almost everyone has had some experience with alcohol, it's a useful way to introduce the issue of substance addiction.

There have been many definitions of alcoholism over the years, and none of them involve things like "drinking alone" or "drinking before noon." Many people are aware that only a minority of persons with alcohol problems wind up as bleary-eyed panhandlers on downtown streets, and that an alcoholic might well be able to hold down a job, pay taxes, and go to services every Sabbath.

In its definition of alcoholism, the National Council on Alcoholism and Drug Dependencies includes *impaired control, preoccupation with alcohol use, continued drinking in spite of adverse consequences,* and *denial.*

All definitions of problem drinking include a person's *loss of control* over their drinking, perhaps the most important part of the definition. A person who drinks when alcohol is available even though he had previously decided he wouldn't is showing a loss of control over his drinking; so is the person who goes to a party intending to have one or two glasses of wine but ends up having seven or eight.

Preoccupation with alcohol means spending more and more time thinking about alcohol and about things like where and how to get it and how to get away with drinking without getting caught. Having availability of alcohol in mind when deciding which friends to socialize with and which parties to go to is a part of this preoccupation. Soon, alcohol is not just a part of social activities but rather the axis around which everything else revolves.

The alcoholic *continues to drink despite adverse consequences* as alcohol begins to replace everything else as the most important thing in the alcoholic's life and becomes the center of his world. No price to pay is too high to use it. The disapproval of loved ones and friends, job problems, legal problems, and even alcohol-related medical problems will not deter the alcoholic from the pursuit of alcohol.

Another important aspect of any definition of alcohol abuse (or any drug abuse) is the alcoholic's denial of the seriousness of his problem with alcohol. *Denial,* when used as a psychological term, means more than just a refutation, or saying "no." Rather, it is a way to manage psychological conflict by simply rejecting the existence of one "side" of the conflict. The alcoholic wants desperately to continue drinking but does not want to think of himself as a problem drinker (and thus, someone who *must* stop drinking). He deals with these opposing sets of desires by denying to himself and everyone else that he has a drinking problem. It's important to emphasize that someone in denial truly believes that what he is denying is not true. The alcoholic in denial believes that he does not have a drinking problem. When the alcoholic says, "I can stop anytime I want to" or "I don't drink any more than my friends do," this is not simply making excuses for continuing with a behavior he knows is a problem. Rather, problem drinkers truly believe the things they tell others about their drinking.

Although alcohol is physically addicting and the withdrawal symptoms of abrupt cessation of heavy alcohol use are potentially fatal, a person can certainly have a drinking problem and not be physically addicted. Persons with severe alcohol use eventually begin to experience blackouts. These are episodes of memory loss that occur after a bout of heavy drinking. They may range from not remembering everything that happened at a party where the individual became intoxicated to not remembering going to the party at all. An important signal of physical addiction is a need to drink daily to prevent feeling "nervous" or "shaky."

Marijuana

In 2008, the National Survey on Drug Use and Health found that 25.8 million Americans age 12 and older had abused marijuana at least once in the year prior to being surveyed. The National Institute on Drug Abuse reported in 2007 that 15.8 percent of people entering drug abuse treatment programs reported marijuana as their primary drug of abuse.

For many years, it was commonly believed that no one became physically addicted to marijuana and that it was therefore a comparatively "safe" drug to get high on. This is because cannabinoids, the active components of marijuana, are absorbed into fatty tissues during use and are slowly released when marijuana use stops, making for a sort of automatic tapering effect. This usually prevents withdrawal symptoms. Studies of marijuana users have demonstrated, however, that chronic marijuana users do indeed develop physical addiction: the development of tolerance to the effects of the drug and withdrawal symptoms when the drug user stops using. In a study in which volunteers were given the same measured doses of cannabinoids daily for four weeks, the volunteers reported that the marijuana seemed to become "weaker" and their high became progressively less intense, demonstrating their development of tolerance to the drug; some developed irritability and sleep problems after the drug was stopped.[4] Other studies have confirmed that persons who use marijuana regularly and then stop completely can develop anxiety and panic, depressed mood, irritability, loss of appetite, insomnia, and physical symptoms such as changes in heart rate and blood pressure, sweating, and diarrhea. Marijuana's reputation as a benign drug is undeserved.

Because these effects develop several days after stopping the drug, users can convince themselves that they are only "self-medicating" pre-existing anxiety or depressive symptoms. A regular marijuana user might say that she uses cannabis to "calm her nerves" when in fact the use is to ward off the development of withdrawal symptoms.

Marijuana abusers have the same problems with loss of control as alcoholics, becoming increasingly preoccupied with the drug and continuing to use despite adverse consequences. As with alcohol, some individuals appear to use marijuana "socially" and maintain control over their use, but many do not.

Stimulants and MDMA ("Ecstasy")

Amphetamines include a group of compounds (of which methamphetamine is the most abused) that are potent stimulants of the central nervous system. "Speed," "crystal meth," and "ice" are street names for these pharmaceuticals that make the user feel alert, energetic, and often elated. A decreased sense of fatigue and increased initiative, motivation, and self-confidence occur. Concentration is enhanced, and there is often an increase in activities and productiveness without need for sleep. Because physical as well as mental performance is enhanced, these drugs are prone to be abused by athletes, students cramming for exams, long-distance drivers, and others who desire to artificially boost their alertness and performance. The effects are brief, however, and users often experience depression and fatigue after only a few hours of amphetamine use that may require several days of recuperation. More long-term use or binges of heavy use over several days usually cause a "crash" into more severe depression, with low mood, fatigue, lassitude, and loss of interest and pleasure in activities—the gamut of symptoms of a depressive illness. Changes in appetite occur, as well as vivid, unpleasant dreams and other sleep disturbances that can take weeks to subside completely.

The parent compound, amphetamine, is one of the stimulant medications used to treat ADHD (amphetamine and a related compound dextroamphetamine are combined in the ADHD preparation Adderall; methylphenidate [Ritalin] is another). Diversion of these drugs from legitimate use is a source of some illicit amphetamines, but amphetaminelike compounds can be easily manufactured in basement laboratories from ephedrine, a related compound found in over-the-counter cold and allergy preparations, along with other fairly easily obtained chemical ingredients.

Recently, a group of amphetamine derivatives, sometimes collectively referred to as *club drugs* or *designer drugs*, have been widely abused. *Ecstasy* is a compound called MDMA (from its chemical name, 3,4-Methylenedioxy-methamphetamine), and a related compound is MDA (3,4-methylenedioxy-amphetamine). A 2000 report stated that nearly two hundred of these drugs have been synthesized and described, mostly in underground labs.[5] A pill that is represented to be Ecstasy may, in fact, be any one of these compounds.

Although MDMA is chemically derived from amphetamine, the molecule has structural similarities to mescaline and is often classified as a hallucinogen like LSD. Unlike LSD, MDMA does not usually cause hallucinations, but as with other drugs in this group, users report feeling that their emotions are deeper and more meaningful and that they achieve profound self-understanding and develop new perspectives and insights about themselves and their relationships. Intense sexual arousal is often noted as well (the reason, perhaps, that MDA has been called the "love drug"). The amphetamine-like euphoria and confidence the drug produces makes these experiences all the more intense and powerful.

The adverse psychological effects are, as might be expected, a combination of those reported to occur with amphetamines and hallucinogens: psychotic episodes, panic, and depression. Reports of several poorly understood sudden deaths in users, psychotic episodes, prolonged depressions, memory impairment, and thinking problems are increasingly seen in the psychiatric and toxicological literature.

Prescription Drug Abuse

In a 2009 study of 332 persons who have borderline personality disorder, nearly half of the respondents admitted to abusing prescription medications.[6] The most commonly abused prescription medications fall into two groups: pharmaceuticals used to treat anxiety symptoms called *benzodiazepines,* and narcotic pain medications, such as OxyContin and Percocet (table 6.1).

Although these two groups of medications are used to treat different types of symptoms—panic/anxiety and physical pain—both can cause sedation and euphoria in higher doses, probably because they operate in similar ways on the brain's pleasure center.[7]

These addictions often begin when an individual is prescribed one of these medications for the legitimate treatment of a medical condition but then goes on to take them in higher doses than recommended, for longer periods than recommended, or both. Benzodiazepine abuse can be especially insidious; these medications are so effective in treating anxiety problems that individuals can quite easily start using them to eliminate *any* problems with anxiety—even the sorts of trivial stresses that we all encounter on any ordinary day. Although not developed to treat anxiety, narcotic pain medications also have antianxiety effects, and people can come to rely on them in the same unhealthy way as with benzodiazepines. Individuals eventually develop tolerance to both types of medications, meaning that higher and higher doses are required to obtain the same anxiolytic effect. At higher doses, problems with physical dependence eventually develop, meaning that stopping, or even cutting down, can cause withdrawal symptoms. The individual needs to keep taking the medication just to feel something approaching normal, at which point she is truly trapped.

Eating Disorders

Eating disorders are a group of psychiatric syndromes that share the common element of distorted eating behaviors. Individuals who have eating disorders may eat too little or too much, but all share a preoccupation with food, calories, and weight that comes to be all-engrossing and pathological, sometimes with dangerous, even deadly consequences.

JENNIFER HAD BLACKED OUT *for only a moment, it seemed, but she was still glassy eyed and quiet when the ambulance arrived. The instructor had whisked the other horrified women out of the aerobics studio and called the club's nurse, who had found Jennifer's pulse to be alarmingly low and was now having trouble getting her blood pressure to register on the BP cuff. When Penny had hiked up the young woman's long sweatshirt to take her blood pressure, she was taken aback by how skinny Jennifer's arm was.*

"Has this girl been sick?" she asked.

"Not that I know of," replied the instructor. "At least not anything serious. She's missed a few classes now and again, but only one or two."

They heard the sirens wailing up the health club's driveway. "Good," thought Penny, "they're here."

She looked down at Jennifer again. "Why are you wearing these heavy sweats for an aerobics class?" she asked. Perhaps the girl had become overheated and fainted.

"I'm always cold," replied Jennifer listlessly.

The studio doors swung open, and three paramedics in sharply pressed blues briskly walked in. The nurse and the instructor sprang back, and Jennifer was on the gurney in seconds. One of the paramedics pumped up the blood pressure cuff that was still on her limp arm and listened intently with her stethoscope. "Sixty-five over zip," she announced. Another paramedic had already pricked Jennifer's finger and squeezed a drop of blood into what looked like a handheld calculator. He read the number that glowed on its little screen. "Her blood glucose is only thirty-seven, Kate." Kate looked down at Jennifer. "Are you diabetic, honey? Do you take insulin?" she asked. Jennifer shook her head weakly.

"What did you have for breakfast today, sweetie?"

"A vitamin pill."

"We're going to start an IV on you." In a moment, Jennifer, the gurney, and the three paramedics were moving toward the door. "We're taking her to Memorial. If you have an emergency contact for her, call them. We might need somebody else to give us her medical history." The room was quiet as the voices of the paramedics died away. Then the siren's wail started up and slowly faded.

Penny turned to the instructor. "Carol, has this woman seemed tired to you? Has she had trouble keeping up with the others in this class?"

"No. Jennifer's always full of energy."

"Do you know anything else about . . ." A sign at the front of the studio caught her eye. "Weight loss?" Penny said. "This is a weight-loss class?"

"Yes, it's been one of our most popular—"

"That girl does not have a weight problem."

"I started the Thursday night group last month, and Jennifer was the first to sign up. I didn't think she looked overweight, but it's hard to tell with those baggy clothes she always wears."

Penny looked thoughtful for a moment, then asked, "Do you ask these women how much weight they want to lose when they sign up?"

"They fill out a form with their current weight and their goal weight. I remember that Jennifer left those questions blank. I just thought she was embarrassed . . ."

Penny wasn't listening anymore, though. She realized that this girl probably did have a weight problem, but not the kind of problem an aerobics class would help with. Jennifer had listed her mother as her emergency contact; Penny noticed that Jennifer and her mother lived at the same address. When she was able to get Jennifer's mother on the phone, she asked about her eating habits.

"They're terrible. I know she's too skinny. Her father and I have begged her to go see the doctor. She never eats with us anymore. I almost think it's better that way because every meal turned into a screaming match. We can't even talk about it around here. Her father gets so mad about it that I worry about his blood pressure getting out of control again."

"Mrs. Andrews," the nurse said slowly, "I think Jennifer might have an eating disorder."

By the time pop singer Karen Carpenter died from anorexia nervosa in 1983, an event that brought eating disorders into the consciousness of most Americans for the first time, physicians had been aware of this mysterious group of psychiatric illnesses for over two centuries. In 1874, the English physician William Withey Gull coined the term *anorexia nervosa* to describe "a morbid mental state" that resulted in extreme weight loss. Gull realized that the weight loss was not due to a bodily illness like tuberculosis or an intestinal disease but was instead the result of "simple starvation."

But it was the French *alienist* Lasègue who first captured the essential elements of this form of the illness: a "refusal of food" that becomes "the sole object of preoccupation and conversation" such that "the circle within which revolve the ideas and sentiments of the patient becomes more narrowed." Lasègue described the disconnect between the patient's appearance and her perception of her appearance and assessment of her nutritional needs: "The patient, when told that she cannot live upon an amount of food that would not support a young infant, replies that it furnishes sufficient nourishment for her, adding that she is neither changed nor thinner." Lasègue also recognized the upheaval the syndrome causes in families and the frustration and powerlessness of the parents of these patients. He noted that the family "has but two methods at its service which it always exhausts—entreaties and menaces."[8]

In the 1980s, it was recognized that self-starvation is not the only serious abnormal eating syndrome. Patients were described, often of normal weight, who binged on huge amounts of food in a matter of hours or even minutes and then caused themselves to vomit what they had eaten. The terms *binge-purge syndrome* and *bulimia nervosa* (or simply *bulimia*) were coined to describe these patients.

More recently, overweight patients who binge but do not induce vomiting or use other means to compensate for their increased calorie intake have been described, and the diagnosis *binge-eating disorder* has been proposed to designate this syndrome.

It's been suggested that perhaps the biggest group of persons with abnormal eating behaviors do not fit neatly into any one of these classifications but have elements of several or shift from one clinical picture to another over time. Abnormal eating syndromes cover a wide range of problems from those with minor health risks to those that are life threatening.

As with substance abuse, the topic of eating disorders is an enormous and complicated one that would easily need a book of its own to cover in any depth. What follows, then, is a brief overview of the main symptoms of the disorders to introduce them and shed light on the interplay between these syndromes and other aspects of borderline personality disorder.

Anorexia Nervosa

The most dramatic and severe of the eating disorders is *anorexia nervosa*. Persons who have anorexia believe they are overweight, even obese, and restrict their food intake to lose weight. Despite their steadily decreasing weight and the emaciated appearance of their bodies, they continue to view themselves as overweight and keep restricting. The name of the syndrome is incorrect in a sense, because the word *anorexia* is a medical term for loss of appetite and does not characterize these persons (except perhaps in the advanced stages of starvation, when their brain functions are abnormal in many different ways). They *fight* their hunger, and after a time, the struggle against their appetite becomes an end in itself, the focus of all their energies.

Individuals with anorexia lose their objectivity about calories and weight as their drive to lose weight takes on a life of its own. Often, the person starts out with a desire to lose what might indeed be extra pounds, but soon she cannot identify or be satisfied with a healthy goal weight. She may identify an initial goal weight of 110 pounds but then decide to lose down to 105 when she reaches that initial goal. At 105, the new goal becomes 100, then 95, and eventually the only goal is to weigh less than the day before—with no end in sight. The person often becomes convinced that if she starts to gain weight, she will lose control of her eating and ability to maintain her weight and become enormously obese. Some people realize they are thin but worry that some part of their body, such as their abdomen or buttocks, is "fat." Eating comes to be viewed as a vice; taking needed nourishment is "giving in."

As others notice the person's increasing thinness with alarm, eating and meals become more and more tense. As Lasègue observed in the families of his patients, "the delicacies of the table are multiplied in the hope of stimulating the appetite; but the more the solicitude increased, the more the appetite diminishes. The patient disdainfully tastes the new [foods] and after having thus shown her willingness, holds herself absolved from obligation to do more."

Persons who have anorexia not only fast but also exercise excessively to lose weight. They may use laxatives and diuretics (fluid pills) to decrease calories and weight. To avoid the stares and comments of others, they dress in baggy clothing that conceals their emaciation.

Eventually the physical consequences of starvation begin to take their toll. Menstruation stops, heart rate slows, and hands and feet become cold as the body attempts to conserve calories. Skin becomes dry, hair may fall out, and the person complains of fatigue and is noted to be listless and lethargic. Dizzy spells and fainting occur. Eventually sodium and potassium imbalances affect cellular functions, heart rhythm abnormalities develop, and the person can die from cardiac arrest.

The consequences of malnutrition on psychological functioning are profound. In a 1945 study, male "conscientious objectors" were placed on a diet that effectively reduced their weight to the level of a person with anorexia. Interestingly, although they had no prior history of wanting to lose weight, they began to have serious consequences. They developed severe depression, diminished judgment, and preoccupation with food, including self-restricting during the re-feeding phase of the experiment. Self-injury also was observed, and one participant cut off three of his fingers with an axe, then reported confusion as to whether it was purposeful or accidental.[9] The results of this experiment highlight the need for addressing malnutrition first in treating patients who have anorexia nervosa. Though internal psychological processes may have caused the behaviors in the first place, psychotherapies (such as trying to understand why the patient has an intense fear of fatness) and attempting to reason with her to eat more are fruitless. The person must be re-fed to a healthy body weight before she will have the cognitive abilities to participate in therapy.

After re-feeding, a lengthy retraining process must occur during which the patient relearns normal eating patterns and changes her feelings about herself, her weight, and her relationship with food and calories. In severe cases, lengthy psychiatric hospitalization is necessary to accomplish this work.

Bulimia

The hallmark of bulimia is binge eating, during which persons eat enormous amounts of food, often sweet high-calorie foods, over a period of an hour or so. Individuals will eat an entire gallon of ice cream at one sitting, dozens of doughnuts, several whole pizzas, candy by the pound—usually stopping only when they are physically incapable of taking in any more food. A binge is a private affair undertaken secretly and alone; food consumption is frenzied, joyless, and obsessive, and the person feels out of control, almost "out of body," while it is happening.

When a person who has bulimia cannot force another bite, she is overcome with disgust and shame at what she has done and seeks a way to rid herself of the calorie load. The vast majority of persons who have bulimia do this by forcing themselves to vomit. This provides them relief from the physical discomfort brought on by the binge and reduces their fear of gaining weight from such an enormous intake of calories. Individuals with bulimia usually stimulate their gag reflex by putting a finger or spoon down the throat in the early stages of their disorder but often become adept at vomiting at will. Those who do not manage this may actually develop a callus on the first knuckle of their finger from the repeated abrasions of their teeth during self-stimulation to induce vomiting. Persons who have bulimia may also misuse laxatives and diuretics to get rid of calories and water weight.

The binge is often an unplanned and impulsive response to some uncomfortable emotional state. As with anorexia nervosa, persons who have bulimia are abnormally preoccupied with their weight and body image and often strictly control their diet and avoid high-calorie foods aside from their binges. However, unlike those who have anorexia nervosa, these persons are often normal weight or slightly overweight.

Persons who have bulimia nervosa are usually impulsive in other areas of their lives and behaviors and often have a history of substance abuse, self-mutilation, and suicide attempts. Many people who have anorexia nervosa have bulimic behaviors, and approximately 40 percent of them have a more prolonged bulimic phase in the course of their illness or recovery.[10]

Physical complications of bulimia nervosa are mostly related to repeated vomiting. Stomach acid erodes the enamel of the teeth and causes sore throat. Repeated vomiting causes fluid imbalances that result in weakness and fainting, and disturbances in sodium and potassium balance can cause heart rhythm problems.

Binge-eating disorder has been proposed as a diagnosis for persons who binge but do not purge, use laxatives, or engage in other behaviors to get rid of the extra calories. As might be expected, these persons are often overweight.

The treatment of bulimia nervosa includes helping the person identify the precipitating factors of a binge, addressing her distorted body image and abnormal attitudes toward food, and teaching her healthy eating habits and alternative ways to cope during periods of emotional distress.

Understanding Eating Disorders

Like substance abuse problems, eating disorders are best understood as complex, self-reinforcing *behaviors* that entrap vulnerable individuals. The challenge to understanding eating disorders is that of comprehending how self-starvation and binging and purging can possibly be self-reinforcing, that is, why some people, on some level at least, are *attracted* to these behaviors in the same way that substance abusers are attracted to alcohol and drug use. It will help to first identify the vulnerabilities that are the "setup" for these behaviors.

Social and cultural factors are important. Eating disorders are seen almost exclusively in industrialized countries where a food shortage is not significant. Western culture's glorification of thinness in females is also an important factor. One need only glance through any magazine marketed to teenagers to see the idealized feminine physique: willowy thin supermodels or buxom but toned and wiry beach beauties—often photographed and touched up in such a way as to make them look even thinner than they are in real life. Surveys show that up to 70 percent of young women in Northern Europe and the United States feel they are overweight even when they are thin or normal in weight. Yet most women simply do not have the genetic endowment needed to look like those they see depicted in magazines, on billboards, and in films and television programs. Adolescent boys feel some of the same pressures, but the emphasis is on being muscular rather than thin. This is one of the reasons why eating disorders are thought to be so much rarer in males (and perhaps why steroid abuse is almost exclusively a problem of men).

There is also something of a class consciousness attached to thinness, exemplified by the popular saying that "a woman can never be too rich or too thin." In contrast to cultures in which food is scarce and plumpness is valued, in cultures where food is plentiful, slimness and the avoidance of obesity is valued and associated with wealth. Being overweight is associated with laziness, poor self-control, and self-indulgence; thinness is associated with good health and self-discipline. Young people constantly see and hear that thin is good and fat is bad, and they incorporate these ideals into their view of what sort of body type is attractive and desirable.

While most individuals are relatively unaffected by this barrage of messages about weight and appearance, a person who doesn't feel good about herself can take it to heart in a serious way. As we mentioned previously, persons who have borderline personality disorder are often tormented with bad feelings about themselves, and damaged self-identity is one of the defining characteristics of the diagnosis. These individuals also fear losing control of life and usually feel ineffective and helpless to affect the outcome of what happens to them. Some become preoccupied with food and weight control to distract themselves from these frightening issues.

When they restrict and experience a weight loss, they often experience a surge of feelings of competence, self-confidence, and control. Complimentary and congratulatory comments from others on their successful weight loss further reinforce weight loss as an admirable goal. Fasting and food preoccupation becomes a "safe place" where they feel in control and know that their efforts will pay off in predictable and measurable ways. The person who has anorexia begins to take pride in her ability to adhere to stricter, narrower, and more abnormal diets and restricts her food intake further and further. Thinness, fasting, and exercise are seen as virtues and eating as a vice. The person becomes intoxicated by her success at losing weight and tries to reach ever more ambitious weight-loss goals.

The 1945 experiment mentioned earlier, in which healthy volunteers went on extremely restricted diets to study the psychological effects of starvation, has shown that continually hungry people begin to think and talk about food constantly, even dreaming about food. As her food intake decreases, a person who has anorexia experiences ever stronger, now physiologically induced food cravings, and she finds that she must work ever harder to keep the weight off. She develops increasingly irrational fears about what would happen if she were to begin eating normally, imagining that her body would balloon to immensely obese proportions if she stopped restricting. More fasting leads to more craving and hunger, which leads to more food preoccupation, more fear of losing control—and this leads to more fasting. A vicious circle develops. The individual has become intensely fearful of eating, but now, fasting is the only way she knows of to deal with feelings of anxiety. There is no escape.

Eventually, malnutrition begins to affect brain functioning. At this point, the person becomes physically incapable of making good decisions about eating or realizing how dangerous a situation she is in. This is the reason that at very low weights, people require hospitalization to accomplish re-feeding.

Persons who have bulimia follow a comparable course. These individuals are affected by the same sociocultural factors regarding thinness and also worry about their weight. They often go on diets that are unreasonable and overly strict, and their initial binges are the results of impulsive and out-of-control eating to quickly alleviate their hunger pangs. Alternatively, the binge may have developed as a means of dealing with depression, loneliness, and anxiety. In either case, binging becomes the coping mechanism and simultaneously the cause of shame, guilt, and disgust. The person starts purging to rid herself of the physical discomfort and calories that result from the binge, but this behavior (and perhaps weight gain that results from binging as well) causes more shame and guilt, precipitating more binging, and another vicious cycle begins.

Unfortunately, food abundance often comes with advanced technology. The Internet, and more particularly social networking, has enabled people who have these eating disorders to join together in a sort of exploded codependent relationship in which the members reinforce each other's abnormal eating behaviors. There are many "pro-ana" (anorexia) and "pro-mia" (bulimia) Web sites. Some groups even wear specific wristbands to identify themselves.

In the treatment of eating disorders, eating behavior and attitudes toward food and body need to be retaught to the patient. She must also learn new ways of coping with uncomfortable feelings and address self-image and self-esteem issues. Many of these individuals also have an underlying mood disorder that fuels the maladaptive coping mechanisms, and that disorder requires treatment in its own right.

Eating Disorders and the Borderline Diagnosis

Clinical research studies indicate that eating disorders are about twenty times more common in persons who receive the diagnosis of borderline personality disorder than in the general population; about one-quarter of persons who have BPD have a serious eating disorder, and twice that have at least some distortions in their attitudes toward food and their eating behaviors.[11]

Why this extraordinarily high percentage? Unfortunately, research has not answered this question definitively. But a number of things about eating disorders and BPD offer clues. We know, for example, that most people who have eating disorders suffer from a mood disorder, a risk factor with a very high prevalence in people with the borderline diagnosis. As far as temperament and personality traits, it has been shown that persons with eating disorders have an elevated neuroticism scale compared with the general population,[12] a finding that characterizes borderline personality disorder as well. As you'll read in the next chapter, persons with the borderline diagnosis frequently have a personal history of childhood trauma (abuse or neglect), which is also known to be a risk factor for later developing an eating disorder.[13] So, as you can see, persons who have BPD frequently have many risk factors for eating disorders as well.

The relationship between eating disorder and borderline personality disorder is likely one of complicated interactions that differ from person to person. It is crystal clear, however, that when they occur together, *both* problems require treatment. As with the combination of substance abuse and mood disorders, treating one problem does not usually make the other go away.

The treatment of severe eating disorders is complicated and requires a team of experts. Severely malnourished individuals are best served in psychiatric hospitals that have a special eating disorders unit and a treatment team that is experienced in treating these disorders. It has also been demonstrated that a specific behavioral treatment for borderline personality disorder (dialectical behavioral therapy, which we will discuss later) can be successfully modified to treat patients who suffer from an eating disorder as well.[14]

CHAPTER 7

Behaviors II

Self-Harming Behaviors and Dissociation

In this chapter, we first talk about a group of behaviors that are extremely common in persons with the borderline diagnosis, behaviors in which the individual intentionally injures or threatens to injure himself. These include cutting behaviors and other forms of self-mutilation as well as the ultimate self-harming behavior, suicide.

Then, we briefly discuss a disconnected, trancelike mental state that has been termed *dissociation*, another behavior sometimes seen in individuals who have borderline personality disorder that provides temporary relief from unbearable feelings.

Cutting and Other Forms of Self-Mutilation

Here are several personal accounts of young women's first episodes of self-mutilation:

I was in the bathroom going completely crazy, just bawling my eyes out, and I think my mom was wallpapering—there was a wallpaper cutter there. I had so much anxiety, I couldn't concentrate on anything until I somehow let that out, and not being able to let it out in words, I took the razor and started cutting my leg and I got excited about seeing my blood. It felt good to see the blood coming out, like that was my other pain leaving me too. It felt right and it felt good for me to let it out that way.[1]

I remember the first time I started cutting myself. I was sitting in the school field at break time and rubbing a piece of glass up and down my arm. It hurt but the pain felt comforting and it focused my emotions on that point of my skin. When I bled it felt like all the bad feelings just flowed out of me.

From then on, it was as if I had found my escape mechanism. I never had to deal with out-of-control panic, fear, anger, rage or vulnerability again. I could just bleed.

By my late teens I was an empty shell. I felt nothing any more, and no one could reach me or hurt me. I lived in a strange, safe, isolated world.[2]

Self-mutilation is deliberate, nonsuicidal self-injury, usually by cutting or burning the body. It is a behavior that evokes horror and disgust and seems utterly irrational. Even suicide is, in a sense, easier to understand: a desire to end one's suffering arising out of a profound hopelessness and despair. The intentional self-infliction of pain and disfigurement is, on the other hand, incomprehensible, at least at first glance. Unfortunately, self-mutilation is not rare, and it has been estimated that "cutters" and other individuals who repeatedly harm themselves number in the millions, affecting about 1,000 persons per 100,000 population per year.[3] The prevalence of this behavior among patients being treated for borderline personality disorder is much higher, reported to be as high as 70 percent in one study.[4] About a third of these patients reported first harming themselves as children (12 years of age or younger), another third started as adolescents (13–17 years of age), and a third as adults (18 or older).[5] Like substance abuse and eating disorders, self-inflicted injury is a multifaceted behavior with no single "cause." Various factors lead to it and cause it to be repeated. Self-mutilation occurs in vulnerable individuals, is precipitated by emotional distress of various types, and is sustained by additional and usually different factors.

Fortunately, these behaviors decrease dramatically over time in persons with the borderline diagnosis. In McLean Hospital's ten-year Collaborative Longitudinal Personality Disorders study, the percentage of patients engaging in self-mutilation decreased from over 90 percent to less than 18 percent (see table 7.1).[4]

As with eating disorders, it's quite a challenge to understand how

Table 7.1 Percentage of individuals engaging in self-harm in a group of patients with borderline personality disorder followed for ten years

Study entry (290 patients)	90.3% (262)
2 years (275)	50.9% (140)
4 years (269)	35.3% (95)
6 years (264)	28.4% (75)
8 years (255)	22.4% (57)
10 years (249)	17.7% (44)

Source: Adapted from Zanarini, M. C., F. R. Frankenburg, D. B. Reich, G. Fitzmaurice, I. Weinberg, and J. G. Gunderson, "The 10-year course of physically self-destructive acts reported by borderline patients and axis II comparison subjects," Acta Psychiatrica Scandinavica 117, no. 3 (2008): 177–84.

self-mutilation can make a person feel better in any way and to identify what feelings draw people to hurt themselves again and again. As with eating binges, episodes of self-mutilation seem to start out with inner tension or distress that gradually builds to a point where it is unendurable. Individuals report that injuring themselves provides an instant relief of this unbearable tension. They compare the relief they experience to "lancing a boil," "popping the lid off a pressure cooker," or "bursting a balloon." The injury focuses frustration and emotional pain in the harmful act, and some persons report a sense of regaining control of their mental state by their self-injury. This sense of relief may last for hours, and the individuals often go into a deep sleep afterward.

This behavior is not suicidal behavior because the persons are not acting out of a desire to end their lives; rather, individuals with this problem report that the behavior gives them rapid, though short-lived, relief from uncomfortable emotional states, including depression, anxiety, and anger. Often, the person feels guilty and ashamed afterward and attempts to conceal what she has done.

The range of self-injuring behaviors is broad. Some people make only superficial skin scratches with their fingernails or pick at skin blemishes. At the other end of the continuum are people who collect razor blades, surgical gauze, and antiseptics and make careful incisions that they cleanse and bandage afterward. Burning with lit cigarettes or heated metal objects is another common method of self-harm. Self-mutilation seems to be a brief, time-limited behavioral syndrome for most (playing out over a period of weeks or months), and only a minority of persons who repeatedly injure themselves develop the sort of addiction to the behavior that can go on for years. Like eating disorders, individuals who self-mutilate appear to be predominantly female.

Why Do Individuals Self-Harm?

The most widely accepted model for explaining cutting and other self-destructive behaviors is the idea that self-injury is a strategy to alleviate acute negative emotions or affective arousal. This reasoning also has the most research to support it.[6] A refinement of this model that specifically applies to persons who have BPD theorizes that early negative environments may teach poor strategies for coping with emotional distress in individuals[7] who also, as we explained in chapters 4 and 5, appear to have a biological predisposition for emotional instability that makes them less able to manage emotions. For them, self-injury is a maladaptive emotion-regulation strategy.

Many persons also say that they engage in these behaviors to keep from feeling numb. We previously discussed how individuals who have BPD are frequently troubled by feelings of profound emptiness and loneliness. They sometimes report feeling unreal or nothing at all, and self-injury may be a way to generate emotional and physical sensations that allow them to feel "real" or alive again.

It has also been proposed that self-injury provides a means of expressing suicidal thoughts without risking death, that is, as a kind of replacement for true suicidal behaviors.

Because this behavior shocks and horrifies others, especially family members, essentially rendering them gasping and helpless, it can be a potent and dramatic way to act out anger and replace fear and depression with feelings of power and control. In a psychiatric research periodical issue devoted to the topic of self-mutilation, the scientific editor, a well-known psychiatrist, wrote in the introduction, "The typical clinician treating a patient who self-mutilates is often left feeling a com-

Table 7.2 Functions of deliberate self-injury examined in the research literature

Function	Description of function
Affect regulation	To alleviate acute negative affect or aversive affective arousal
Feeling generation	To end the experience of feeling unreal, outside their body, or nothing
Antisuicide	To replace, compromise with, or avoid the impulse to commit suicide
Interpersonal boundaries	To assert one's autonomy or a distinction between self and other
Interpersonal influence	To seek help from or manipulate others
Self-punishment	To express anger toward oneself
Sensation seeking	To generate exhilaration or excitement

Source: Adapted from E. D. Klonsky, "The functions of deliberate self-injury: A review of the evidence," *Clinical Psychology Review* 27, no. 2 (2007): 226–39.

bination of helpless, horrified, guilty, furious, betrayed, disgusted and sad."[8]

The same kinds of social factors that influence the development of eating disorders may be at work in self-harming behaviors as well. In 1992, *People* magazine published excerpts from a biography of Princess Diana that revealed not only her eating disorder behaviors but also episodes of cutting herself. Just as the glorification of thinness and the societal pervasiveness of dieting lead increasing numbers to attempt to lose weight and traps a few of them into eating disorder behaviors, the glamorization and romanticizing of self-injury in the famous may facilitate initial episodes of cutting.

The treatment of self-mutilation resembles that of eating disorders in that the person must be persuaded to give up a behavior that, however perverse, is powerfully addictive. Therapy to identify the sources of uncomfortable emotional states and to learn alternative ways of coping with them is extremely important. Like eating disorders and substance abuse problems, treating repetitive self-mutilation is complex and requires intensive, long-term multidisciplinary therapy, preferably by specialists in the area of treating these problems. In chapter 10, we will discuss in detail a proven therapeutic technique for treating patients who engage in repetitive self-mutilation, a technique called dialectical behavioral therapy (DBT). Originated by Dr. Marsha Linehan at the University of Washington in Seattle, DBT was developed specifically to treat individuals with repetitive self-harming behaviors and repeated suicide attempts, and focuses on helping the patient identify and interrupt the thinking and emotional processes that lead up to an episode of self-mutilation.

Suicidal Behavior

Borderline personality disorder is the only psychiatric disorder in the DSM that has "repetitive suicidal behavior" as one of its diagnostic criteria, indicating how extremely common this symptom is in people who have BPD. Research indicates that over three-quarters of persons with the borderline diagnosis make a suicide attempt, and approximately 10 percent of patients with this diagnosis die by suicide.[9] Many of these persons make repeated suicide attempts, and a significant percentage have suicidal thoughts almost continuously. Studies indicate that emotional instability (comparable to the five-factor trait "neuroticism") is most closely associated with the whole range of suicidal behavior.[10] Individuals who eventually succeed in completing suicide have been found to have a higher number of psychiatric hospitalizations and prior attempts. A history of childhood sexual abuse confers additional risk for suicidal behavior, and another risk factor that shows up in the studies of completed suicide in persons with borderline personality disorder is a diagnosis of substance abuse.

Many studies have attempted to tease out differences between more serious suicidal behavior (where the person unambiguously wanted to die and used a more lethal means in their attempt) and attempts that were highly ambivalent or used a method of low lethality (an overdose of only a few pills or on a medication with low toxicity). The problem with this approach is that persons who make a suicide attempt are nearly always ambivalent on some level, and these behaviors occur while they are in such a distraught psychological state that asking them to analyze their "intent" or "reasons" at the time may not be terribly reliable.

Nevertheless, when persons who have made some sort of suicide attempt, whether of low lethality and highly ambivalent intent or the opposite, are asked about their mental state just prior to the attempt, many of the same reasons emerge as those that precipitate nonsuicidal self-harm, such as cutting behaviors.

Escape from intolerable mental anguish is the most frequent reason given; in one study, 86 percent of individuals who had made a serious suicide attempt stated that the main reason for the attempt was to get relief from emotional pain.[11] This same study found that about half of the subjects also reported some interpersonal factor underlying their behavior, such as an attempt to communicate the severity and intensity of their distress to someone else, to get someone to change her attitude or to act differently, or simply as a cry for help. This very maladaptive communication strategy may be one of the only ways to send these messages that the person who has borderline personality disorder can muster: "A single dramatic threat or act effectively circumvents the normal and lengthy process of negotiating support and reassurance from others—a relationship experience that many [of these patients] may have rarely encountered in their own family experience."[12]

These attempts are usually triggered by some immediate traumatic event, most frequently an interpersonal problem such as arguments with significant others and family members, or incidents in which the individual felt disappointed, angry with, or abandoned by someone close to them.[13]

From what you have read in this book so far, it should not be difficult to understand why persons who have BPD are so troubled by suicidal thinking and behaviors. Their problems with damaged identity make them especially sensitive to rejection—they feel so bad about themselves continuously that rejection, even the most trivial, seems like a confirmation of their feelings of worthlessness. In a sense, they don't have any "self" to fall back on for support. Their tendency to react strongly and quickly with negative emotions, which they cannot adequately modulate on their own, means that their emotional reaction to perceived rejection escalates out of control fast, like a runaway train careening down a hill. Add impulsiveness and an inability to self-soothe to this potent mix, and you truly have a recipe for disaster. If the individual has an addiction as well, the well-known inhibition-lowering effect of alcohol or drugs makes things much worse, as does any coexisting mood disorder.

In figure 7.1, we've taken a highly regarded model of adolescent depression and modified it to explain the processes that lead to a suicide attempt in persons with borderline personality disorder. This multifactorial model proposes that suicidal thinking originates from an underlying psychiatric disorder, but that it smolders under the surface until some stressful event precipitates more active consideration of suicide, and then actual suicidal behavior is either facilitated or inhibited by a combination of mostly external factors.

The cascade begins with some psychiatric disorder or disorders that research has shown puts people at high risk of suicidal behaviors, in this case, the problems with intense and unmodulated negative emotions that are part of the borderline diagnosis, and any additional risk factors, such as a mood disorder or substance abuse problem.

The suicide attempt is precipitated in these vulnerable individuals by a *stress event*, such as the breakup of a relationship or simply a recent distressing or humiliating argument. The stress event leads to an acute emotional crisis with the development of extreme anxiety, dread, and hopelessness. A sense of inner tension and agitation builds, and the individual feels compelled to "do something."

At this point external factors either facilitate or inhibit suicidal behavior. Being or feeling isolated and unable to reach out for comfort or support appear to be facilitators. The availability of a supportive, trusted influence such as a family member, a close friend, or a therapist to help soothe and decompress the situation would be inhibitors. A strong religious belief about the sinfulness of suicide would inhibit, whereas living in a culture where suicide is seen as an acceptable solution to problems would facilitate.

Other suicide facilitators include opportunity and access factors,

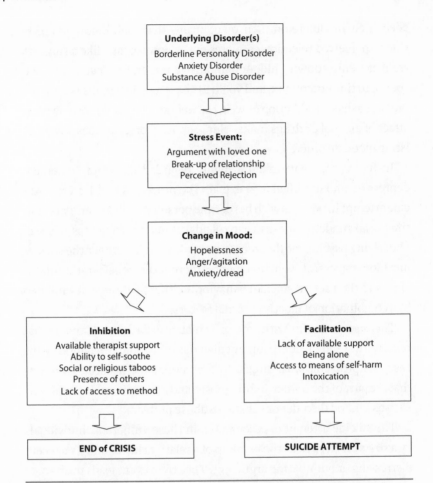

Figure 7.1. A model for suicidal behaviors in borderline personality disorder.
Adapted from D. Shaffer and L. Craft, "Methods of adolescent suicide prevention," *Journal of Clinical Psychiatry* 60, supp. 2 (1999): 70–74.

such as being alone at home and the availability of a highly lethal suicide method like access to a gun. Perhaps the ultimate facilitating factor is intoxication of some type. Numerous studies indicate that a substance abuse diagnosis greatly increases the risk of suicide, and most persons who kill themselves have alcohol in their bloodstream when they do so.

Efforts at suicide prevention need to focus on every step of the process that leads to suicide: identifying the psychiatric disorder and getting the individual into treatment, which teaches personal coping skills to deal with crises and to modulate emotions as well as providing the external therapeutic support these persons need.

Dissociation

The term *dissociation* is used to refer to a variety of psychiatric symptoms that share as their common element some form of disturbance in a person's awareness of and mental connection to his surroundings. These experiences aren't as bizarre as you might think on first hearing about them. Perhaps you've had the experience of driving down a highway you knew extremely well to a familiar destination when you started thinking about something so compelling that you momentarily lost awareness of your surroundings, briefly driving on "autopilot," only to realize a few moments later that you don't remember driving the last mile or so. Such an experience of "getting lost in your head" is a mild and not unusual dissociation experience. Dissociative symptoms are most common in persons who have experienced some type of severe psychological trauma. Among the worst and most distressing of these symptoms are flashbacks, where something in the environment triggers an involuntary recollection of a traumatic event that is so intense and vivid that the sufferer feels as though he is actually re-experiencing it, complete with feelings of intense panic, helplessness, and horror. There are, however a whole range of symptoms between these two extremes (table 7.3).

For several decades, military psychiatrists have become increasingly aware of the significant numbers of combat veterans who are troubled so much by these symptoms that they are impaired in their functioning and relationships. The term PTSD (post-traumatic stress disorder) is now familiar to almost everyone. A 2001 study found that, after going through extremely physically and psychologically stressful military survival training (that included stresses such as sleep deprivation, semistarvation, exposure to extremes of heat and cold, and social isolation), over 95 percent of healthy young military recruits reported some of the dissociation symptoms listed in table 7.3.[14] One of the important findings from this study was that soldiers who had previously experi-

Table 7.3 Dissociative symptoms

Things seem to move in slow motion.

Things seem unreal, as if in a dream.

Feeling separated from what is happening, as if watching a movie or a play.

Having a sense of watching things from outside one's body.

Feeling as if one were watching the situation as an observer or a spectator.

Having a sense of being disconnected from one's body.

The sense of one's own body seems changed.

People seem motionless, dead, or mechanical.

Objects look different than expected.

Colors seem diminished in intensity.

Things seem to happen very quickly, as if there were a lifetime in a moment.

Things happen that one is unable to account for later.

People and objects appear far away or unclear, as if one were looking at the world through a fog.

Source: Adapted from the Clinician-Administered Dissociative States Scale

enced a traumatic experience, especially a life-threatening experience (such as a physical assault or severe motor vehicle accident), reported substantially more symptoms. This would suggest that individuals who have suffered a traumatic event are sensitized by the experience and more vulnerable to these symptoms if they experience traumatic events later in life.

Many studies have demonstrated that persons who have borderline personality disorder frequently suffer from various distressing dissociative experiences. One group of researchers reported that about half of the persons who had BPD that they interviewed described "clinically significant" symptoms of dissociation.[15]

Dissociative "Disorders"

Several psychiatric syndromes that share some of the symptoms we have just discussed have been known collectively as *dissociative disorders*. We discuss them here because for many years, they were a source of controversy and notoriety, garnering much attention in the general media. The most prominent of them is what had been called *multiple personality disorder* (now referred to as *dissociative identity disorder*), in which an individual seems to develop additional "personalities," each with an independent identity. Various other syndromes in this group are likewise characterized by some disturbance of identity or memory, including *fugue* and *amnesia* syndromes, where the individual appears to forget who she is for days to months or spends time in a trancelike state that can last long enough for her to travel to another community and even establish a new identity. It was thought that these problems were also related to trauma, especially childhood sexual trauma, and supposedly occurred when an individual somehow isolated traumatic memories into split-off "pieces" of herself that developed into new identities.

These diagnostic categories are no longer accepted by most mainstream psychiatrists, and there is considerable doubt as to whether these "disorders" really exist as clinical entities. Most of the early publications on these persons were little more than vivid descriptions by enthusiastic practitioners of their own patients. As other researchers started to study these individuals, it became apparent that, for the most part, they were suggestible persons who had developed "alter personalities" only after getting into treatment with a therapist who suggested that "multiple personality disorder" explained their emotional misery. The research journal *Dissociation* ceased publication in 1997 (though it has now been succeeded by the *Journal of Trauma and Dissociation*), and published reports on these problems in peer-reviewed scientific literature have slowed to a trickle. Much of what is being published is critical and discrediting of the diagnoses.[16]

A large percentage of the patients who received (and, unfortunately, are still receiving) diagnoses of "dissociative disorders" have borderline personality disorder. However, these diagnoses are best thought of as clinical constructions created by overenthusiastic practitioners in patients desperate for answers, professional support, and new ways to cope with unbearable feelings. As one expert observed:

> Patients with borderline personality disorder are in tremendous emotional pain and are eager to understand the factors that led to this pain. Patients also long for close, emotionally intense, even exclusive relationships with their therapists. The combination of a therapist who is sure of what went wrong in a patient's life and who is offering a simple, albeit emotionally charged solution to a complex problem, and a patient who is in enormous pain and who is longing for attention and closeness often leads to . . . negative outcomes.[17]

While some persons who have BPD experience dissociation symptoms for brief periods, the idea that they have dissociative episodes that go on for days or weeks, or "alters," and that these problems constitute independent disorders is no longer accepted.

Dissociation Symptoms in Borderline Personality Disorder

Dissociation symptoms in persons with the borderline diagnosis are seen predominantly in those who have a history of significant psychological trauma. The McLean study that we have frequently referred to throughout these chapters found that a history of one of four specific types of psychological trauma has the most significant association with dissociative symptoms. These were (1) inconsistent treatment by a caretaker, (2) sexual abuse by a caretaker, (3) witnessing sexual violence as a child, and (4) an adult rape history.[18]

We will discuss in more detail in the next chapter the significance of a trauma history for individuals who have BPD. Here we will simply say that "zoning out" and other symptoms such as those listed in table 7.3 appear to be acute reactions to the overwhelming pain these persons experience when an event, or even a set of feelings, triggers an emotional overload from re-experiencing the fear and horror of a past trauma.

The treatment of these symptoms emphasizes helping individuals bring themselves back into control by focusing on the here and now, and by observing and participating in the present moment, practices called mindfulness skills.[7]

CHAPTER 8

The Life Story

Childhood Experiences, Development, Trauma

In this chapter, we discuss how *what the person has experienced* contributes to the problems of borderline personality disorder. In many ways, this may be the most familiar way of thinking about psychological issues and psychiatric disorders. Sigmund Freud, arguably the first scientist to develop a comprehensive theory of mental functioning, emphasized this method of reasoning nearly to the exclusion of all others in his efforts to explain human behavior. Freud's legacy is our acceptance of the idea that our experiences, especially early childhood experiences, have a powerful effect on us, making important contributions to how we think about ourselves and the world, how we relate to others, and how we cope and adjust to setbacks that occur later in life.

Freud developed his ideas during a time when practically nothing was known about the biological workings of the brain; therefore, he developed a theory of mind that does not depend at all on any knowledge about brain functioning. This is, of course, the great shortcoming of his method. He assumed that the human mind at birth was a *tabula rasa*, a blank slate, and that everything about how the mind functions was caused by our environment and experiences in the world. We now know that many psychiatric illnesses, such as schizophrenia and mood disorders, are caused by disruptions to the normal biological functioning of the brain. Freud developed theories to explain how experiences, including experiences during infancy, led to the development of these problems, too—theories that we now know are quite inadequate. Nevertheless, Freud's ideas have led to the development of an enormous body of knowledge over the last one hundred years or so, knowledge that forms the basis of the approach that psychotherapists use to help patients.

One of Freud's fundamental ideas is that our experiences *always* affect us in some way, often in ways we are only dimly aware of, and that they therefore play a role in our mental life. Another fundamental idea is that childhood experiences are especially important and have powerful effects, and that the experiences and early relationships we have with our parents are the most important of all, having the most long-lasting effects on us. While there are many aspects and details of Freud's theories that have not proved to be very helpful in understanding human behavior—not even most psychiatrists can give you an accurate definition of "Oedipus complex" anymore—and others we now know are just dead wrong, his fundamental ideas have truly stood the test of time.

Childhood Experiences and the Borderline Diagnosis

One of the corollaries to these ideas about the importance of childhood experiences is that there are a few basic requirements for what we might call a "healthy" childhood environment, and that childhood environments that deviate too far from these basic requirements increase the chances of long-term problems in psychological functioning. This is another idea that can accurately be said to have stood the test of time. It is well established that how we are treated as children is important in shaping how we think about ourselves, and that as little children, we learn about how healthy relationships work from our relationships with the important people in our lives, usually our parents.

From these assumptions, it follows easily, then, that in trying to understand persons who have borderline personality disorder, those who have tremendous relationship problems and appear to have a damaged self-identity, researchers early on started looking at the childhood experiences of the individuals.

When they did so, researchers found that many of these people had experienced some significant loss in childhood or had a strained and conflicted relationship with their parents. Numerous studies found that individuals who had borderline personality disorder were much more likely than individuals who had other psychiatric problems to have experienced the loss of a parent through death, divorce, or a severe illness that required prolonged hospitalization—up to three-quarters of people who had BPD in one early study.[1] Those in these earlier studies who had BPD were also more likely to report strained or distant relationships with a parent.

The results of these studies led researchers to start asking about extremes of childhood difficulties, and many studies followed in the 1990s that examined the prevalence of physical and sexual abuse during childhood in persons who had BPD. These studies tended to be more scientifically rigorous than the ones from prior decades, making diagnoses more carefully, collecting information about childhood in more standardized ways, comparing the findings in individuals with borderline personality disorder to those in individuals with other personality disorders, other forms of mental illness, and healthy control subjects. In many of these studies, great effort was taken to eliminate researcher bias by making sure that the clinician making psychiatric diagnoses for the study did not know the subject's childhood history, and that the researcher collecting the childhood history didn't know the diagnosis of the subject being interviewed. Again, it was found that persons with the borderline diagnosis were much more likely to report abuse during childhood than those with other psychiatric diagnoses. A study that compared the childhood histories of over 300 patients with the borderline diagnosis who required treatment on an inpatient psychiatric unit to those of 109 patients who had other personality disorders found that almost two-thirds of the patients with borderline personality disorder reported childhood sexual abuse, compared with about one-third of the patients with other personality disorders.[2]

It's important that we point out two significant facts about the data on trauma history and borderline personality disorder: (1) not all people with the borderline diagnosis have experienced sexual trauma in their lives, and (2) we know from other research that *most* individuals who have been victims of childhood sexual trauma *do not* go on to develop borderline personality disorder. We will return to these findings later.

Other studies examined more subtle problems with parenting in persons who have BPD and have consistently found that they were significantly more likely to report having a caretaker withdraw from them emotionally when they were children. Individuals reported inconsistent parenting, such as being praised or punished in unpredictable ways, perhaps due to a parent's own problems with mental illness. They reported experiences in which parents tended to deny or discount their thoughts and feelings as children, or treated them as a friend or confidant or even a parent.

A theory of psychological development called *object relations theory* emphasizes the role of our parents in how we think about ourselves and others in our lives, suggesting that the patterns we develop during childhood in response to parenting experiences affect relationships later in life. This approach proposes that adverse parenting experiences cause the child to develop an identity or self-image of themselves as "bad" or "helpless" and to tend to see other people as powerful but often punitive. This is thought to lead individuals to initially *idealize* important people in their life and have unrealistic expectations of others' ability to protect and nurture them, and when those expectations are not met, to feel betrayed, helpless, and mistreated—or perhaps even deserving of punishment.

Inconsistent parenting experiences are, of course, found in the backgrounds of many persons, most of whom do not go on to develop borderline personality disorder. Why some children are more adversely affected by these experiences is not entirely clear, but it has been proposed that extremes of temperament or perhaps genetically determined problems with emotional regulation are risk factors for these problems. Dr. John Gunderson, who has done much of the groundbreaking research on BPD, put it this way: "Borderline [personality disorder] arises out of a history in which abusive experiences join other factors to help shape enduring aspects of character."[3]

These findings and theories have found their way into the thinking of Dr. Marsha Linehan of the University of Seattle, who uses the term *invalidating environment* to describe the commonality of ways in which this wide variety of adverse experiences contributes to the symptoms and problems of these individuals. Dr. Linehan developed dialectical behavioral therapy, one of the most successful treatment approaches for these patients. We discuss this treatment approach in chapter 10, where we also go into more detail about the proposed pathway from these childhood experiences to borderline symptoms. The basic idea is that in an invalidating environment, the "pre-borderline" child's identity, worth as a person, and feelings are consistently ignored or dismissed in some way by those who are responsible for being supportive and nurturing. Sexual abuse is obviously the most egregious violation of a child's worth and feelings, but the research shows that even subtle forms of caregiver rejection, emotional absence, or inconsistent parenting can cause problems in children who are temperamentally less able to modulate feelings and who tend to react more easily and more negatively to emotional stresses.

Borderline Personality Disorder and PTSD

Studies that have taken a more nuanced look at the connection between childhood experiences and BPD have demonstrated that the more childhood adversity a person has had, the more severe and debilitating his borderline symptoms. There is evidence that the more severe symptoms of borderline personality disorder, such as paranoid thinking, extreme problems with self-destructive behaviors, and dissociation are seen primarily in individuals with significant sexual or physical abuse histories. One study showed a direct statistical association between the severity of sexual abuse history and the severity of dissociation symptoms.[4] This has led some to propose that borderline personality disorder is better thought of as a complicated and chronic form of post-traumatic stress disorder (PTSD). At the least, there is definite overlap between the symptoms and the histories of persons who have BPD and persons who have PTSD. It has also been shown that a significant proportion of individuals with the borderline diagnosis also suffer from the full array of PTSD symptoms. This overlap bears further discussion.

It has been recognized for many decades that soldiers who had witnessed horrific events and been through life-threatening experiences during wartime sometimes developed a debilitating set of symptoms that included things like flashbacks to the event, when they felt and acted as if they were back in combat, as well as a more general tendency to become emotionally over-reactive and unstable in their emotional lives. *Shell shock* and *battle fatigue* were earlier terms for these problems; following the Vietnam War, the term PTSD was coined, and research on these problems began in earnest.

It soon became clear that this syndrome was not limited to combat veterans but could occur after exposure to any severely traumatic event. Studies of victims of natural or manmade disasters, and victims of physical or sexual assault, found that clinically significant PTSD symptoms occur in some proportion of individuals who have been exposed to a whole variety of traumatic experiences. The proportion varies widely and appears to be somewhat related to the severity of the trauma. A 2010 study found that about one in ten Norwegian tourists who survived the 2004 East Asia tsunami developed PTSD, while approximately one in five lower Manhattan residents developed PTSD following the 2001 terrorist attack on the World Trade Center. A prior history of exposure to unusual stress, as well as pre-existing difficulties in coping, increases the risk of developing PTSD following a severe trauma.

PTSD is diagnosed when the syndrome develops following traumatic exposure in an individual who had not previously been troubled by its symptoms. The diagnostic issues become much more complicated when the trauma occurs over a prolonged period or during childhood, when the symptoms can be more subtle—both factors are characteristic of childhood abuse.

It has been proposed that the intense psychological reactions that persons with the borderline diagnosis develop in response to conflict in a relationship and perceived loss represent a re-experiencing of childhood abuse or neglect or simply family conflict or inconsistent parenting. It has also been suggested that the dissociative experiences and paranoid thinking that these individuals experience in reaction to rela-

Table 8.1 Summary of DSM-IV diagnostic criteria for post-traumatic stress disorder

The person has been exposed to a traumatic event in which both of the following were present:
- The person experienced, witnessed, or was confronted with an event that involved actual or threatened death or serious injury, or a threat to the physical integrity of self or others.
- The person's response involved intense fear, helplessness, or horror.

The traumatic event is persistently re-experienced in one (or more) of the following ways:
- recurrent and intrusive distressing recollections of the event, including images, thoughts, or perceptions
- recurrent distressing dreams of the event
- acting or feeling as if the traumatic event were recurring (includes a sense of reliving the experience, illusions, hallucinations, and dissociative flashback episodes, including those that occur on awakening or when intoxicated)
- intense psychological distress at exposure to internal or external cues that symbolize or resemble an aspect of the traumatic event
- physiological reactivity on exposure to internal or external cues that symbolize or resemble an aspect of the traumatic event

Persistent avoidance of stimuli associated with the trauma and numbing of general responsiveness (not present before the trauma), as indicated by three (or more) of the following:
- efforts to avoid thoughts, feelings, or conversations associated with the trauma
- efforts to avoid activities, places, or people that arouse recollections of the trauma
- inability to recall an important aspect of the trauma
- markedly diminished interest or participation in significant activities
- feeling of detachment or estrangement from others
- restricted range of affect (e.g., unable to have loving feelings)
- sense of a foreshortened future (e.g., does not expect to have a career, marriage, children, or a normal life span)

Persistent symptoms of increased arousal (not present before the trauma), as indicated by two (or more) of the following:
- difficulty falling or staying asleep
- irritability or outbursts of anger
- difficulty concentrating
- hypervigilance
- exaggerated startle response

tionship problems are basically the same as those experienced by persons who have PTSD when exposed to something that reminds them of their traumatic history. Table 8.1 gives the DSM criteria for PTSD.

Many studies demonstrate that a significant proportion of persons who have borderline personality disorder can also be diagnosed with PTSD. One study of patients being treated on an inpatient unit in a psychiatric hospital found that 58 percent of them also had the full syndrome of PTSD.[5] Since this study was done on hospitalized patients who would have had much more severe symptoms and problems in functioning, it is representative of more severely ill patients; other studies have found PTSD to be far less common in persons who have BPD.

So how to explain these overlaps in symptoms and the tendency for these two problems to coexist more often than would be expected? On one extreme are the proposals that borderline personality disorder is best thought of as a complex form of PTSD, in which the disorder is complicated by histories of abuse over prolonged periods, starting in childhood. But it has been amply demonstrated that childhood trauma is neither necessary nor sufficient to result in the development of borderline personality disorder, effectively disproving such a direct causal relationship.

Another idea is that individuals who have borderline personality disorder are more likely to experience trauma during adulthood because of their impulsivity and tendency to have conflicted and volatile relationships. That is, PTSD symptoms in persons who have BPD are due to repeated traumas experienced in adulthood. At least one study investigated this possibility using a sophisticated statistical technique called *path analysis,* which attempts to elucidate likely pathways to a disorder, and failed to demonstrate such a relationship.[6]

Finally, there is the possibility that individuals who have a history of adverse childhood events are at higher risk of being in that proportion of individuals exposed to trauma in adulthood who develop PTSD; that is, problems during childhood somehow sensitize an individual to trauma and increase the likelihood of developing PTSD following later traumatic exposure. The research literature on PTSD in combat veterans is supportive of this idea; even subtle family dysfunction during childhood increased the risk of developing PTSD in a group of marines returning from combat duty.

We are left with the somewhat unsatisfying explanation that the symptom overlaps between borderline personality disorder and PTSD, and the tendency for these problems to co-occur in many people, is because of intertwining but inconsistent causal factors.

As is the case with borderline personality and mood disorders, addiction, and many of the other problems we have discussed in the last four chapters, biological vulnerabilities, temperamental predispositions, and life events all interact to result in a broad range of difficulties in emotional life and in pathological behaviors like addiction, eating disorders, and other self-harming behaviors.

Life Events in Adulthood

Research indicates that, in addition to having more adverse childhood experiences than others, persons who have borderline personality disorder tend to encounter more stressful life events as their life progresses compared with other people and have more difficulty coping with them.

A study from Australia asked nearly a hundred individuals receiving psychiatric treatment about the number of important and potentially stressful life events they had experienced in the previous six months.[7] These were not necessarily traumatic events; even events usually thought of as positive can be stressful: getting a new job, getting married, having a child, and so forth, are usually stressful. Leaving no stone unturned in their efforts to assess even the most trivial of life events in these patients, the researchers also asked them to fill out a questionnaire called the Hassles and Uplifts Scale. This questionnaire lists several dozen areas of life (important areas like children, health, and job security as well as mundane areas like yardwork and car maintenance) and asks the subject to indicate how much of a hassle or how much of an uplift each item was for them. Last, the subjects answered questions about how well they were functioning at work, in their relationships, and in several other areas. For the analysis, the subjects were divided into three groups whose results were compared: patients who had borderline personality disorder, patients who had some other personality disorder, and patients who had a serious psychiatric illness such as major depression or bipolar disorder, but who did not have a personality disorder.

The results of this study indicated that persons who had BPD experienced more significant life events than any other group of patients tested. As might be predicted, the particular events tended to center on relationship issues (a breakup or divorce, arguing more with family members, but also getting married or engaged). The subjects with a BPD diagnosis also reported experiencing more hassles and fewer uplifts in day-to-day life than the other subjects, and experiencing their hassles as more intense than others reported. On the scale that measured daily functioning, the subjects who had BPD showed the worst level of functioning compared with the other two groups, especially, as might be predicted, in the domain of interpersonal functioning.

Using a sophisticated statistical method called *regression analysis*, which can distinguish co-occurring factors that might be causing an illness or problem, the authors found that the diagnosis of borderline personality disorder, the number of stressful life events, and the perceived intensity of day-to-day hassles all *independently* predicted lower levels of functioning in these subjects. That sounds much more arcane than it really should; let us put it another way: in this study, having borderline personality disorder predicted a lower level of functioning, but also predicted a greater number of stressful life events, which, in turn, predicted lower functioning, as did more intense hassles, which . . . well, you get the idea. Basically, in persons who have borderline personality disorder, their problems with coping, the stressful life events that they encounter, and their intense reactions to those events all feed on each other in a vicious cycle that perpetually interferes with the person's functioning—not to mention his chances for happiness.

Fortunately, however, specialized treatment for borderline personality disorder is quite successful in interrupting this cycle. In part 4 of this book, we will discuss those treatments one by one and hope to persuade you that, far from being hopeless, borderline personality disorder is becoming more and more recognized as an eminently treatable psychiatric problem, usually with an excellent prognosis.

III

Treatment

CHAPTER 9

Treating the Disease

We will now start discussing the treatment of borderline personality disorder. As you learned in the last section of the book, this disorder is a complex collection of interacting symptoms and behaviors with many types of causes. We told you that one way to unpack this complexity is to view the disorder from four different perspectives and talk about disease (what the person *has*), about personality traits and temperament (who the person *is*), the unhealthy behaviors that the individual develops attempting to cope (what the person *does*), and how the individual's life experiences have affected the ways in which she feels and behaves (what the person has *encountered*). In this first treatment chapter, we review treatments for problems that are rooted in biological functioning, problems that can be best understood as disease states with biochemical causes that can be successfully treated with medication to correct or compensate for anomalies in biological functioning.

KATE HAD THOUGHT *that coming to terms with the diagnosis of borderline personality disorder would be the hardest part. She had begun to see how messed up her life had become and, in a way, always had been. It was true that a lot of it wasn't her fault, although there were some things that she could change and take a hold of. Her boyfriend could still be a jerk some of the time, but she had started to figure out that the more she let go, the happier she was. Still, she continued to have really good days and really bad days; nothing even had to happen to set her off—some days she just got up on the wrong side of the bed and everything got worse from there.*

She was discussing this with her psychiatrist when he dropped a huge bomb in the middle of the room—"Have you ever thought about taking medication?" Of course she had—she had friends on pills who said they could help you relax. She'd even taken a couple for a flight once. But she soon found out that this wasn't exactly what he meant. "I think that you could really benefit from a medication that could help stabilize your mood swings, maybe bring you more toward the middle. One of the oldest and most widely used medications is lithium, and it's still one of the best . . ." She stopped listening. Does he think I'm crazy? "There's no way I'm putting that poison into my body—my mom used to take that and ended up with her kidneys giving up, and she was still no better from it," she announced. "I mean, a little something once in a while to relax, maybe, but lithium?"

Psychiatry has come a long way since the time of Freud. There are now many pharmacological options in addition to psychotherapy among our therapeutic tools. The unfortunate reality is that the idea of taking psychiatric medication carries a lot of emotional baggage. Being prescribed a daily medication can make people feel that

- there is something drastically wrong with them
- they can't possibly fix it themselves without medication because they are ineffective or weak
- they'll never be normal

Many people carry these sorts of stereotypes; we have had patients who pay out-of-pocket for their psychiatric medications because they don't want psychiatric medications to show up on their insurance record, or who insist on having close relatives pick up the medication for them so that they won't be seen in the pharmacy. Occasionally, they do not even tell their regular family physician about their psychiatric medications for fear of being labeled as a "crazy" patient—but not sharing this information can lead to dangerous medication interactions.

The facts about psychiatric medications are far different. They can augment (rather than replace) psychotherapy, making this form of treatment much more successful, much faster, than it would otherwise be. Medications are not meant to be disempowering or to make you feel like you are a slave to a pill; rather the opposite—they are meant to help restore control so that a person can reach her full potential. Just as with the treatment of diabetes or high blood pressure, medications can often diminish symptoms to the point of total resolution—and can be life saving.

What follows is a summary of the types of medications used in treating borderline personality disorder and the evidence for their efficacy (or lack thereof). We have, for the most part, left out discussions of dosing and side effects, not because these are unimportant issues, but because an adequate discussion would at least double the number of pages in this book. Also, this is a discussion that a person needs to have with her doctor at every appointment, part of the monitoring process that is so important for successful medication treatment. Suffice it to say here that there is always the possibility of adverse reactions to any medication; some are common, many are rare. Most will be temporary inconveniences that quickly fade as the medication starts to work; some, however, are serious enough to warrant discontinuing the medication. Fear of adverse effects should not be a reason to avoid effective medications; this disorder is often much more disabling than any medication side effects. Also, remember that the rundown on a medication's side effects that the pharmacy gives you is a list of *possible* side effects, not a list of what you should *expect* to experience.

We have used several very different sources of information for this chapter. They include the treatment guidelines of the American Psychiatric Association[1,2] and of the British National Institute for Health and Clinical Excellence[3] as well as the Cochrane systematic review of clinical trials of pharmacotherapy for borderline personality disorder from the Cochrane Collaboration, an international organization that commissions statistical analyses (called meta-analyses) of only the most rigorously designed and executed clinical studies of treatments.[4] We also discuss other options supported by the research literature.

What Do Medications Treat in Persons with Borderline Personality Disorder?

Studies that have attempted to determine the effectiveness of medications in borderline personality disorder can be difficult to interpret. Some studies have been done on persons with the borderline diagnosis who also have the mental illnesses that we know frequently co-occur in this group of people, illnesses like bipolar disorder, major depressive disorder, and post-traumatic stress disorder (PTSD). Other studies have been done after excluding persons who meet diagnostic criteria for these disorders. Some have argued that trying to draw conclusions from both types of studies is therefore a case of "apples and oranges."

Obviously, if a person who has BPD also has one of the illnesses we mentioned, then effective treatment for the other problem will be beneficial. But does that mean his borderline personality symptoms have gotten better? Of course, one could argue, what difference does it make? Better is better. But the question remains: if a person suffers from borderline personality disorder but does *not* appear to have one of these illnesses, should he be prescribed medication? The short answer is: we don't know for sure. Problems in the way many studies are conducted (often referred to as "methodological" problems) on persons with the BPD diagnosis prevent anyone from drawing definite conclusions.

The National Institute for Health and Clinical Excellence (NICE), Great Britain's equivalent of the National Institutes of Health (NIH) in the United States, has taken what might be the most conservative position: that strict interpretation of the research literature supports medication treatment *only* for what are called *comorbid* conditions, meaning mental illnesses like bipolar disorder or PTSD that co-occur in persons with BPD. The authors of the NICE recommendations are not convinced that existing studies justify prescribing medication to patients unless one of these illnesses can be diagnosed with confidence. The report of the international Cochrane Collaboration, on the other hand, side-steps the issue of which symptoms are of comorbid conditions and which are core symptoms of borderline personality disorder and simply evaluates a person's relief of symptoms and improvement in functioning while taking medications. They report that the research literature supports the idea that medications can alleviate many problems common in persons who have BPD (symptoms like aggressiveness, angry outbursts, impulsivity, and problems in interpersonal functioning) and essentially leave aside the issue of which symptoms are comorbid and which are core.

The authors of the NICE recommendations took the Cochrane authors to task for this, insisting that available studies have just too many methodological flaws to draw strong conclusions. "We do not recommend drug treatment *other* than for the treatment of comorbid disorders," they state, adding, "More good-quality evidence is required" (emphasis added).[5]

The American Psychiatric Association (APA) takes a more pragmatic middle ground (as do we), essentially blending these two approaches. Many, perhaps most, persons who have borderline personality disorder do indeed have a comorbid condition like bipolar disorder, and treating this problem appropriately is immensely important in helping them to recover. It's unfortunately beyond the scope of this book to survey all treatments for every possible comorbid condition. To adequately review treatment for mood disorders, PTSD, panic disorder, and all the other various illnesses that many persons with the borderline diagnosis also have would require several more books. Instead, we've listed several good resources on the treatment of these comorbid conditions in appendix A.

Like the APA, we think it's reasonable to review the research that has been done evaluating *symptom*-based treatment with medication, and we do so in the remainder of this chapter, reviewing the use of antidepressant agents for the treatment of depressive symptoms and mood stabilizers for treating problems with emotional modulation. Both types of drugs have also been recommended as treatment for the severe impulsivity of borderline personality disorder. Last, we review the evidence that a fairly new group of medications, with the rather confusing and misleading label *atypical antipsychotic,* can be helpful for symptoms that involve distortions of thinking.

Antidepressant Medications

One of the cardinal features of borderline personality disorder is a collection of feelings of emptiness, anger, sadness, and worthlessness,
symptoms that also characterize a major depressive episode. It's not
surprising, then, that mental health professionals have thought that
antidepressants may improve symptoms in people who have borderline
personality disorder.

Although it's been abundantly clear that antidepressants are effective for people who have depressive disorders like major depressive
disorder and dysthymic disorder, it's been difficult to show definitively
that these medications benefit persons with the borderline diagnosis
over and above those beneficial effects. Nevertheless, several studies indicate that some antidepressant medications may help with the
depressive symptoms all persons with BPD experience (that is, not only
those with comorbid depressive disorders) as well as with symptoms
such as uncontrollable anger, aggressiveness, and impulsivity.[6]

Selective Serotonin Reuptake Inhibitors

The medications called selective serotonin reuptake inhibitors (SSRIs)
are so commonly prescribed in medical practice and discussed in the
media that it is almost impossible not to be familiar with them (table
9.1).

Researchers have been studying the brain for many decades seeking
a biochemical correlate of depression. Much of the earliest work showed
that older antidepressant medications (which we will discuss below)
increased the amounts of certain chemicals in the brain responsible
for transmitting signals between brain cells (called *neurotransmitters*).
Decades earlier, Julius Axelrod, a scientist at the National Institutes
of Health, had found that when he injected small amounts of neurotransmitters into animals, 30 to 40 percent of the chemicals were taken
up by the brain cells that normally release them, leading him to propose
that there must be tiny molecular "pumps" in brain cells responsible
for doing so. He later demonstrated that antidepressants do indeed

Table 9.1 Selective serotonin reuptake inhibitors

Pharmaceutical name	Brand name(s)
Citalopram	Celexa (Cipramil)*
Escitalopram	Lexapro (Cipralex)
Fluoxetine	Prozac, Serafem (Erocap, Fluohexal, Lovan, Zactin, and others)
Fluvoxamine	Luvox
Paroxetine	Paxil, Paxil CR[†] (Aropax, Seroxat, and others)
Sertraline	Zoloft (Altruline, Aremis, Gladem, Besitran, Lustral, Sealdin, and others)

*Names in parentheses are brands marketed outside the United States.
[†]Slow-release preparation

increase levels of neurotransmitters in the brain by inhibiting these molecular reuptake pumps.[7]

Later research implicated one particular neurotransmitter called *serotonin* as especially important in depression. This led pharmaceutical companies to develop new drugs that could increase the amount of serotonin in the brain, without increasing other brain chemicals that were thought to be responsible for the various unpleasant side effects common with the older antidepressants. The search was on for drugs that would be specific (*selective*) to *serotonin* and work by blocking (or *inhibiting*) the *reuptake* molecules that pump serotonin back into cells.

The first *selective serotonin reuptake inhibitor* had many side effects unrelated to its mechanism of action and never made it onto the market. The second SSRI was fluoxetine, which was eventually marketed as Prozac.[8] Not only did this medication have drastically fewer side effects than older antidepressants, it had fewer interactions with other medications and was safer if taken in overdose. More SSRIs were subsequently developed and have been shown effective in treating depression as well as some of the symptoms of borderline personality disorder noted above.

Nevertheless, there has been controversy surrounding the use of SSRIs. When first discovered, they were considered almost a magic bullet for the treatment of depression. They were safe and effective enough that doctors began prescribing them to all sorts of patients, including those who felt they were a little too sad, who were somewhat more anxious than other people, or who were just not at the top of their game.

In August 2004, an article in the *London Observer* (with the title "Stay Calm, Everyone, There's Prozac in the Drinking Water") revealed that the British Environmental Agency had detected tiny amounts of the medicine in the water supply of some towns, having been excreted in the urine of persons in upstream towns that released treated sewage into waterways. Unfortunately for this class of medicines, this same year, worry that SSRIs could lead to an increase in adolescent suicides emerged. Both these issues have been largely resolved. SSRIs turn out to be among many other pharmaceuticals and household chemicals that can be detected in the drinking water of many communities around the world. The amounts, however, are in the range of parts per *trillion*, and although all the implications are not known, this exposure has never been demonstrated to be harmful to humans.

When the United States Food and Drug Administration (FDA) reviewed the issue of suicide and SSRIs, they found that no completed suicides had occurred among nearly 2,200 children treated with SSRI medications in clinical trials, although a small percentage (approximately 4 percent) of adolescents taking SSRI medications experienced suicidal thinking or some form of behavior, about twice the rate of those taking placebo. The FDA issued a warning about this finding and recommends close follow-up for patients, especially young patients, who start on any antidepressants.

Tricyclic Antidepressants

Tricyclic antidepressants significantly predate the SSRIs (table 9.2); the first published report on a tricyclic appeared in 1958.[9] They are prescribed much less frequently now, largely because of their long list of possible side effects. For persons who do not respond to the newer medications, however, the tricyclics remain a useful group of medications. Tetracyclic antidepressants (so called because they have four carbon rings in their structure instead of three) are similar to the tricyclics and include trazodone and mirtazapine (Remeron). The available stud-

Table 9.2 Tricyclic antidepressants

Pharmaceutical name	Brand name
Amitriptyline	Elavil
Amoxapine	Asendin
Clomipramine	Anafranil
Desipramine	Norpramin
Doxepin	Sinequan
Imipramine	Tofranil
Maprotiline	Ludiomil
Nortriptyline	Pamelor
Protriptyline	Vivactil

ies on these medications in borderline personality disorder predate the availability of the SSRIs.

In the 1980s, studies on the use of these medications for the treatment of the depressive and suicidal features of persons who have borderline personality disorder first appeared. The results of these studies have been variable. One group studied the effects of amitriptyline versus haloperidol (an antipsychotic) and placebo over four years on inpatients who had borderline personality disorder. They found that amitriptyline was superior to placebo in treating depressive symptoms and hostility, and that it significantly improved self-control. It was also effective on the associated symptoms of depersonalization, paranoia, obsessive-compulsiveness, helplessness, hopelessness, and worthlessness.[10] On the other hand, the closely related tricyclic desipramine was *not* found to be better than placebo in treating depression, anger, and suicidal behaviors when it was compared with lithium and placebo in outpatients who had borderline personality disorder and a low level of comorbidity with mood disorders.[11] Some authors believe that this group of medications might actually be harmful for persons who have BPD, causing what they called "behavioral toxicity"—an increase of symptoms such as impulsivity, aggressive behaviors, paranoia, and suicidal intentions.[12] Little research has been carried out on tricyclics in the past several decades because their use has been eclipsed by the SSRIs. The evidence for use of tricyclic antidepressants in persons who have BPD is, at best, mixed, and they should be used with caution, if at all, unless of course they are needed for an otherwise treatment-resistant major depression.

Monoamine Oxidase Inhibitors

Monoamine oxidase is an enzyme in the brain that breaks down neurotransmitters such as histamine, dopamine, norepinephrine, epinephrine, and serotonin. By blocking this enzyme, more of these chemicals are available to the brain, which (it is believed) is the mechanism by which monoamine oxidase inhibitors (MAOIs) alleviate depression (table 9.3). These medications were actually discovered by accident, when physicians were looking for more efficacious medicines for tuberculosis.[13] They have been thoroughly studied in depression and are known to be quite effective, although they have a significant side-effect burden.

There have been many studies of MAOI effects on borderline personality disorder; again, however, the studies predate the availability of the much safer and easier to take SSRIs. One study from the late 1980s compared phenelzine (60 mg/day) and imipramine, a tricyclic antidepressant (200 mg/day), in outpatients with depression and borderline personality disorder. Improvement was reported by 92 percent of patients administered phenelzine compared with 35 percent of patients administered imipramine.[14] A further five-week study in 1993 showed efficacy of phenelzine over haloperidol and placebo in measures of depression, borderline symptoms, and anxiety,[15] but a follow-up sixteen-week study by the same authors showed no statistically significant benefit.[16] At best, studies have shown a trend toward improvement in depressive symptoms and anger in patients who have borderline personality disor-

Table 9.3 Monoamine oxidase inhibitors marketed in the United States (2010)

Pharmaceutical name	Brand name
Phenlezine	Nardil
Tranylcypromine	Parnate
Selegiline transdermal	EmSam

der. Much more research is needed before this could be recommended as a standard treatment, and as with the TCAs, there has not been research interest in this group of medications for several decades. That said, however, MAOIs can be "miracle drugs" for some people with severe, treatment-resistant mood disorders that no other medications have been able to help.

There are two forms of monoamine oxidase in the body, MAO-A and MAO-B. Until recently, the MAOIs used to treat depression were active in blocking MAO-A. In addition to its activity in the nervous system, MAO-A is also present in the lining of the intestine. This is because a number of naturally occurring substances in various foods are close enough chemically to the neurotransmitter norepinephrine to need deactivation before they are absorbed into the bloodstream. The importance of this becomes clear when we tell you that another name for norepinephrine is adrenaline. Tyramine, an amino acid that has adrenaline-like effects on blood pressure and heart rate, is present in high enough concentrations in some foods to cause dangerous cardiovascular problems in persons on the older MAOIs (phenelzine and tranylcypromine). Several pharmaceuticals, including the ingredients of many over-the-counter remedies, also have adrenaline-like effects. People taking MAOIs therefore need to observe certain dietary restrictions and, even more important, scrupulously read the labels of any over-the-counter medication they are considering—or better yet, consult their pharmacist before taking any pharmaceutical they buy over the counter. MAOIs also interact with other medications that are prescribed or commonly used in emergency rooms for various problems. People taking MAOIs must be sure to inform all their treating physicians of this fact and should consider wearing an alerting bracelet that can communicate to ER personnel that they are taking an MAOI should they be brought into an emergency room after an accident or sudden illness that may impair their ability to communicate with physicians.

Recently, a pharmaceutical that blocks primarily MAO-B, the other form of MAO in the body, has been developed. MAO-B is present almost entirely in the brain and is not involved in blocking tyramine absorption in the intestine. The big advantage of an MAO-B inhibitor over an

MAO-A inhibitor would be that persons taking it wouldn't have to be on a special diet. This drug, called selegiline, has actually been used for the treatment of Parkinson disease for several years. There were early attempts to use it as an antidepressant, but the required doses were so high when taken in pill form that selegiline affected both forms of MAO (A and B); that is, the specificity for MAO-B is lost. This meant that persons taking it would still need to watch their diet for sources of tyramine. Then someone came up with the idea of making a selegiline patch. The patch, whereby the drug is absorbed through the skin rather than taken orally, turns out to have two important advantages. First, because it is more directly absorbed into the bloodstream, the drug can be given at a low dose and maintain its specificity for MAO-B. Second, since it doesn't travel though the intestine, it doesn't affect the MAO-A located there as much. Both these facts mean the selegiline patch is an easier MAOI to take with fewer side effects and less worry about tyramine-rich foods.

Because of these issues, MAOIs are most often prescribed to persons who have failed to benefit from other antidepressants. Occasionally, an MAO inhibitor is taken with another antidepressant. This must be done with extreme care and close monitoring because interactions between MAOIs and other antidepressants can be dangerous. Among other possibilities, it can lead to a dangerous excess of neurotransmitters in the brain, a condition known as *serotonin syndrome*, which, if untreated, can require hospitalization and even lead to death.

Antidepressants in Persons Who Have Borderline Personality Disorder

Many persons who have borderline personality disorder take antidepressant medications because many of them also have major depressive disorder. Should patients with a borderline diagnosis who do *not* also suffer from a depressive illness be prescribed them? The British NICE report answers this question with an unequivocal "No," and we tend to agree. A 2008 American survey of medication studies noted, "The research literature . . . appears to suggest a need for a shift from antidepressants to anticonvulsant [mood stabilizers] and atypical antipsy-chotics" for the treatment of borderline personality disorder.[17] We will discuss these two groups of medications next.

Mood-Stabilizing Medications

We have previously discussed the overlap between the problems of persons who have borderline personality disorder and the symptoms of bipolar disorder. There has long been interest in assessing whether medications effective in treating bipolar disorder might benefit persons with the borderline diagnosis. There is really only a subtle difference between the abnormal mood changes seen in bipolar disorder and the mood modulation problems seen in borderline personality disorder. In bipolar disorder, moods have a life of their own, changing unexpect-edly, often randomly, and getting "stuck" in depressed or manic mode for days, weeks, or even months at a time. Sometimes, the diagnosis of bipolar disorder is quite clear: sustained periods of unexplainable lows and highs with all the associated features of the illness—sleep, appetite, energy, concentration, and self-attitude changes—all point to bipolar disorder and make the decision to start medication straightforward.

In borderline personality disorder, the moods aren't so much ran-dom and unpredictable as they are easily triggered and over-reactive; the problem is with mood modulation:

> I have hair trigger explosions of intense feelings . . . I feel so excited about doing something it's as if I could conquer the world then a couple of hours later it just seems like a load of [nonsense]. I love people one minute and then hate them and want to hurt them the next. Likewise, I can fall in love with someone almost instantaneously then be repulsed by them in a matter of hours. I can be abusive then feel terrible remorse and fear being abandoned.[3]

The two kinds of problems are tremendously difficult to distinguish from each other, and often the only way to know if a mood stabilizer will help is to take one for a time and gauge the benefit or lack thereof.

The term *mood stabilizer* is generally applied to any agent that has both antimanic and antidepressant properties. Despite the indubitable efficacy of these medications in treating bipolar disorder, there really isn't any readily apparent commonality in their biological activity—no common chemical pathway through which they all work to treat bipolar disorder. All these medications, regardless of the precise mechanism by which they do it, appear to enhance the ability of brain cells to function through what have been called *neuroprotective* mechanisms.

The older mood stabilizers, lithium and valproate, have not been studied extensively in persons who have borderline personality disorder without comorbid bipolar disorder, and because of their significant side-effect burden, they are not prescribed much to persons without bipolar disorder. There is a bit more evidence to recommend lamotrigine (Lamictal).

Lithium

The first medication used to treat bipolar disorder, which continues as the gold standard of treatment, is lithium. This medication is the simplest of all therapies, an element that is taken out of the ground, stabilized by mixing it with carbonate or citrate to make a salt, and put into a pill. It was first used to treat psychiatric conditions by John Cade in 1949, who noted that it had a calming effect on animals. He went on to administer it to ten patients with manic symptoms and noted remarkable improvements in all of them.[18]

Though the efficacy of lithium in bipolar affective disorder (for manic episodes, depressive episodes, and long-term maintenance) is well established, there is only one trial of lithium in individuals who have borderline personality disorder, and that one had only ten subjects and was not placebo controlled.[11] Lithium appeared to bring about a decrease in self-mutilation and in symptoms of irritability and anger, but the small number of subjects and lack of placebo group make these results questionable.

Valproate (Depakote)

Another medication used frequently in persons who have bipolar disorder is valproate (Depakote), which was developed as an antiepileptic medication. It was used in France as early as 1963 and only came to the United States as a drug for epilepsy in 1978. The mechanism of action in treating epilepsy is to increase a certain neurotransmitter in the brain that reduces the excitability of neurons. Thus, like lithium, valproate appears to help persons with bipolar disorder through neuroprotective mechanisms.

As with lithium, there is only scant evidence for the efficacy of valproate in the treatment of borderline personality disorder. The trials are small and have many methodological problems; they have been done in groups of patients with and without comorbid bipolar—in one trial, all the patients in the placebo group dropped out before the study was completed. Most practitioners conclude that valproate may have a role in helping people who have borderline personality disorder, but it has a heavy side-effect burden, and for this reason, it is rarely prescribed except to individuals who have bipolar disorder.

Lamotrigine (Lamictal)

Lamotrigine is a relatively new antiepileptic medication that has been used to treat bipolar disorder for about a decade. (The FDA approved it for treatment of bipolar disorder in 2003.) It appears to reduce the amount of excitatory neurotransmitters in the brain, suggesting that like other mood stabilizers, it acts to protect neurons. The first study of lamotrigine in persons who had borderline personality disorder appeared in 1998 and was a one-year trial that showed promising improvements in overall functioning as well as decreases in sexual impulsiveness, substance abuse, and suicidal behavior.[19] A 2004 analysis of the records of patients who had bipolar disorder and borderline personality disorder treated with lamotrigine showed that these patients had improvement in impulsivity and mood lability.[20]

As of this writing, there are two placebo-controlled trials of lamotrigine in individuals who have borderline personality disorder. Of note, in both studies, anyone who had bipolar disorder was excluded from joining, and although only a little over fifty subjects were in the two studies combined, both indicated significant benefits in borderline symptoms. One study investigated the effect of lamotrigine on anger,[21] and the other on the rapid shifts of mood that are called mood lability.[22] Both studies showed positive results from lamotrigine, which, combined with lamotrigine's favorable side-effect profile, offers hope that more and larger studies will be done on persons who have borderline personality disorder and suggest that this drug may be effective for some symptoms of the disorder.

Atypical Antipsychotic Medications

In the 1930s, a group of pharmaceutical compounds called phenothiazines were synthesized in Europe and were found to have antihistamine and sedative properties. In the early 1950s, two French psychiatrists carried out several clinical trials using one of these drugs to treat highly agitated patients suffering from schizophrenia. They discovered that in addition to its quieting and sleep-promoting effects, these medications made the hallucinations and bizarre delusional beliefs of many persons with schizophrenia practically disappear. Phenothiazines, in other words, had a specific effect on the cluster of symptoms usually referred to as *psychotic* symptoms, and thus the name for this group came about: *antipsychotic medications.*

In the 1990s, a new group of antipsychotic medications was introduced that had a much improved side-effect profile (table 9.4). These agents are called *atypical antipsychotic medications* because in addition to the effectiveness for psychotic symptoms of their predecessors, they are also active at serotonin receptors and therefore have significant effects on mood. Their label, "antipsychotic," has become something of a misnomer, because their use in mood disorders is at least as important as their use in psychotic disorders such as schizophrenia, perhaps even more so.

This group of medications has turned out to be highly effective in

Table 9.4 Atypical antipsychotic medications marketed in the United States (2010)

Pharmaceutical name	Brand name
Aripiprazole	Abilify
Asenapine	Saphris
Clozapine	Clozaril
Olanzapine	Zyprexa, Zydis
Paliperidone	Invega
Quetiapine	Seroquel
Risperidone	Risperdal
Ziprasidone	Geodon

treating mood disorders, both major depressive disorder and bipolar disorder, and therefore many persons who have borderline personality disorder take them for these comorbid problems. Because they are effective mood stabilizers for bipolar disorder, they have also been evaluated for the treatment of the severe mood instability characteristic of persons with the borderline diagnosis. Also, since they are effective in treating psychotic symptoms, they have been evaluated for the treatment of the quasi-psychotic distortions of thinking that some people experience:

> Sometimes it seems like people are sneering and laughing at me all the time and [that] attractive women look at me like they are murdering me with their eyes. Other times it is as if I am invisible. At times I hate everyone and everything. Ideas about who I am and what I want to do fluctuate from week to week. My perspectives, thoughts and decisions are easily undermined by what other people think or say and I often put on different voices to fit in. I am never satisfied with my appearance, but then I am never satisfied *per se*—perfect is not even perfect enough.[3]

In both cases, the results have been encouraging. In one study, aripiprazole (Abilify) was found to have both significant effects in the reduction of the "core" borderline symptoms of anger, psychotic symptoms, impulsivity, and interpersonal problems, as well as on depression and anxiety. There have been six trials comparing olanzapine (Zyprexa) with placebo; among these were two large studies including approximately three hundred participants each. They found significant effects for the reduction of affective instability, anger, and psychotic symptoms. There were also statistically significant benefits for the reduction of anxiety.[4] Studies like these informed the author of a review paper, who stated, "The research literature . . . appears to suggest a need for a shift from antidepressants to anticonvulsant [mood stabilizers] and atypical antipsychotics" for the treatment of borderline personality disorder.[17]

Many of the available atypicals have not yet been studied for the treatment of individual who have BPD; many atypicals that are used in other countries are not yet available in the United States; and several more are in the pharmaceutical development pipeline. With so many encouraging results already in, more studies will surely be undertaken to determine how these medications can best be used to treat borderline personality disorder.

Antianxiety Medications: Some Words of Caution

In 1959, a new medication for anxiety was introduced, chlordiazepoxide (Librium), and four years later, a related compound, diazepam (Valium). These were the first of a new class of medications called benzodiazepines. Soon after their appearance on the market, they all but replaced other forms of antianxiety medications, largely because they are much safer.

It is estimated that 10–15 percent of the American population will take a benzodiazepine in a given year. These medications are used to treat all types of anxiety, including panic attacks, as well as other symptoms related to anxiety, like insomnia. As might be expected, they are not infrequently prescribed to persons who have other disorders characterized by prominent anxiety symptoms, including major depression, bipolar disorder, and yes, borderline personality disorder.

The effectiveness of these medications is both their greatest advantage and the biggest worry regarding their use. One professor at Johns Hopkins likens taking a benzodiazepine tablet to having "a very dry martini." This is actually not far from the truth—the therapeutic actions and effects of this class of medications is so close to that of alcohol that they are given to patients in the hospital to prevent or treat alcohol withdrawal symptoms. Unfortunately, they have the potential to be just as addictive.

One of our patients described how she was able to quit drinking only after her physician had prescribed alprazolam (Xanax) for her to take, "to deal with my anxiety." Only later did she realize that she had been using and abusing Xanax just as she had alcohol, but by that point she had become so addicted that she had to go through a medical detoxification before she could stop. Also like alcohol, these drugs cause people who take them on an ongoing basis to develop tolerance (requiring higher and higher doses to achieve the same effect) as well as sedation and sometimes a loss of behavioral control usually referred to by the term *disinhibition*.

Because benzodiazepines are so extremely effective in lessening a distressing but common psychological experience, anxiety, the unwary easily find themselves reaching for the pill bottle to deal with normal everyday anxieties. People can become less and less able to tolerate any anxiety at all and, because of the tolerance these drugs cause over time, find that they "need" higher and higher doses to give them the relief they have come to expect. This is a setup for psychological and physiological dependence on the drug—essentially an addiction. Once a person is dependent on a benzodiazepine, abruptly discontinuing the medication can cause a withdrawal syndrome similar to alcohol withdrawal, a problem so potentially dangerous as to occasionally require treatment in a hospital.

These problems are quite easy to avoid by using these medications for short periods and only at recommended doses.

There have not been many trials on the efficacy of benzodiazepines on borderline personality disorder, but those that have been done have typically produced negative results. One double-blind, placebo-controlled study of sixteen female outpatients showed that the benzodiazepine alprazolam (Xanax) actually increased suicidal thinking and was no better than a placebo for treating depressed mood, aggression, anger, interpersonal sensitivity, and even anxiety.[23] The authors suggested that alprazolam had significant negative consequences in these patients: "We found a significant worsening of serious dyscontrol in patients taking alprazolam compared with those taking placebo. It was necessary to terminate four of the alprazolam trials early because of the severity of the dyscontrol . . . [one patient] threw a chair at her child [although she] had no history of physical violence toward the child . . . [another] patient who cut her neck had no previous episodes of self-mutilation. The serious dyscontrol that occurred with alprazolam seemed rather typical for them, but was more severe, frequent, or unpredictable."[24] In a study of people addicted to or dependent on benzodiazepines, subjects with a diagnosis of borderline personality disorder had the most problems getting off them.[25]

In summary, benzodiazepines can be effective at producing sleep and reducing anxiety. They are best reserved for short-term use to relieve acute anxiety that is expected to resolve (during the occasional plane flight, presurgical worry, or uncomplicated bereavement). However, persons who have borderline personality disorder are prone to have an exacerbation of their core disease features (suicidality, impulsivity, aggression, emotional dysregulation) rather than a reduction in these symptoms. Additionally, these individuals may be more prone to become addicted to these medications and have a more difficult time getting off them. Extreme caution must be exercised when prescribing these medications for anyone; they are probably best not prescribed at all to persons who have borderline personality disorder.

THE USE OF MEDICATIONS to treat psychiatric conditions is a relatively recent development and is one of the most important changes in the field of medicine. Sometimes the right medications can literally make the difference between life and death, between institutionalization and freedom. For people who have borderline personality disorder without any comorbidities (major depression, bipolar disorder, or others), the evidence for their use is less clear. Further investigation is likely needed before there can be a definitive answer. Each individual must have a unique conversation with her own physician about which, if any, medications may help treat her condition. This conversation must of course include a discussion of any and all possible side effects and how they could affect the person's life. None of these medications should be used without thorough consideration. However, for some people, the right medication may mean the difference between a happy, fulfilling life with stable relationships and one hardly worth living.

CHAPTER 10

Treating the Behaviors

Often, the problem *behaviors* of the person who has borderline personality disorder are the most dangerous for the person and the most distressing to family members. Aggressive verbal or even physical behaviors toward those loved ones, unstable relationships, self-mutilating behaviors like cutting, and threats of or attempts at suicide are common features of this diagnosis.

Addressing coexisting biological factors (such as a mood disorder) with prescription medications is one helpful strategy. It's useful to think of the problems that medications treat (depression, anxiety, unstable mood) as the fuel that feeds these raging behavioral difficulties. You may have noticed that the outcome markers in the studies mentioned in the previous chapter (that is, what was measured to determine whether a given treatment was successful) are usually most focused on behaviors (aggression, suicide attempts) rather than feelings (depression, anxiety, etc.). One reason for this is that behaviors are easier to measure than changes in feelings, but another is that the researchers usually considered the behaviors to be the single most important focus of treatment.

However, depriving the behavioral fire of some of its fuel with medications doesn't necessarily extinguish the flames, or prevent occasional dangerous flare-ups. In these individuals, behaviors like cutting have a strong tendency to become habitual, automatic responses to stress, especially interpersonal stress. Since no amount of medication will eliminate these stresses, the person must learn how to stop unhealthy behavioral responses before they get started, learn how to interrupt them when they do, and ultimately prevent them entirely. This involves developing new coping skills, a treatment that doesn't come in pill form.

Stages of Change

Understanding the reasons for disordered behavior does not, all by itself, lead to the ability to stop. If drinking alcohol or cutting is the person's only reliable coping mechanism, understanding *why* that is doesn't really help. No treatment can totally eliminate stressful situations, difficult phases in relationships, depressed feelings, or anxiety. Everyone will always have these things in the course of living, and we will always need to cope with them. Treating a behavioral problem is a matter of learning how to stop a familiar, ingrained, but self-destructive coping behavior and substituting a healthier, more constructive way of coping. It is learning how to change what one *does*.

The most important prerequisite for the successful treatment of behavioral disorders is the individual's acceptance of the need to stop the disordered behavior. This starts with recognizing that the behavior is not working and needs to be given up. This is often the most difficult step. We discussed denial in a previous chapter, a person's ability to convince himself that something staring him in the face simply isn't true. Unless the person overcomes denial and accepts the need to change, treatment to change behavior can't even get started.

One way to conceptualize the process of recognizing the need to change behavior is outlined in the *transtheoretical model*, more commonly called the *stages of change* model.[1] It was initially developed specifically to define the thought patterns and process of behavioral change in smoking cessation but has become a frequently used model to discuss all disorders of behavior. This model proposes that all individuals who successfully change an unhealthy behavior pass through several stages in the process of change in a highly predictable way (see figure 10.1).

The first phase is called the *pre-contemplative stage*. In this phase, individuals are fully engaged in the disordered behavior and have no real intention of stopping or engaging in treatment. They are enamored by whatever advantage the behavior serves (getting high, being thin, etc.) and have little or no appreciation of its negative consequences and dangerousness.

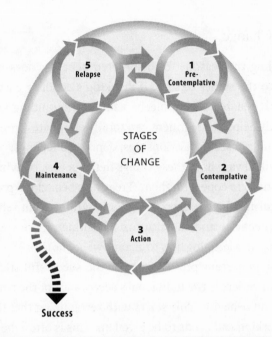

Figure 10.1. Stages of behavioral change. People make behavioral changes in stages, moving clockwise through the cycle from *pre-contemplative* (not accepting the need to change) to *maintenance* (maintaining the behavioral change). Many slip backwards (counterclockwise in the cycle) on their way to recovery, and many suffer a full relapse, progressing from maintenance to the pre-contemplative phase, and needing to go through the cycle another time, even multiple times, before achieving *success*.

The next phase is known as the *contemplative stage*. At this point individuals begin to see that their behavior has at least some negative consequences—to themselves and their health, or to their loved ones. They are beginning to think there might be some advantages to stopping the behavior, and they take some steps to at least investigate what that might entail. They have made no commitment to stop, but they are at least somewhat open to the possibility of stopping. This is one of the most important phases in the cycle, because it is an important place to intervene. People can be stuck here for some time: they may fear the difficulty of stopping, feel uncertain about putting together a plan, or just be "waiting for the right time." This can sometimes be as far as a person gets in the process of change, and it can be a torturous time in their lives; they now see the negative results of their actions but are still powerless to stop.

The third phase is known as the *action stage*. Individuals take steps to implement a plan to stop their negative behavior. This is also a crucial stage in the process—if the loss of the behavior's positive effects or the return of the negative feelings the behaviors were meant to prevent (gaining weight, emotional pain) outweigh developments, individuals may quickly give up on their plan and move back to the contemplation phase. They need a lot of support, empathy, and strong encouragement to keep on track and continue in treatment.

If the action individuals take leads to cessation of the behavior, they enter the *maintenance stage*, in which they continue to abstain from negative behaviors and have coping mechanisms and support in place to do so. As with the action phase, individuals may need a great deal of support to remain committed to abstinence. This can be particularly important as their situation improves and the prior negative consequences of the behavior recede. It is easy to see how seductive thoughts like "just one more time" or "I can handle it now" can sneak in.

One important and unique aspect of stages of change philosophy is that it incorporates the concept of relapse and sees it as a common next phase that many individuals move into. The *relapse stage* is seen not as a failure, but as simply the next phase in the cycle. Many people, when initially trying to stop negative behaviors, will have one (or many) relapses. Seeing this relapse as failure encourages the person to give up, see the process as too hard, and go back to their old ways. Rather, this concept sees it as a nearly inevitable consequence of having a behavioral disorder and understands that people are frequently seduced to revert back to their old ways when they become stressed, or, conversely, when they are quite happy and "let their guard down."

Many people cycle through the stages several times before they have distanced themselves enough from the problem behavior—for which they have substituted healthy coping mechanisms and now have broad and deep support systems—that even maintenance is no longer necessary, and they exit the cycle.

The Talking Cure: Psychotherapy

The word *psychotherapy* comes from the Greek words *psychē*, meaning "breath," "spirit," or "soul," and *therapeia* or *therapeuein*, "to nurse" or "cure." Though first used to describe psychoanalysis, the elaborate and intensive talking treatment developed by Sigmund Freud, it now generally denotes any form of nonpharmacological therapy employed to treat psychological distress.

Freudian psychoanalysis focused on making patients comprehend the workings of their own minds and the meaning behind their actions, with the assumption that understanding these meanings would naturally lead to a change in these actions. Though effective for many patients, progress could take years and depended on an intensive (four to five hours weekly) course of treatment.

Later practitioners modified psychoanalysis to be more short term and efficient but still focused on illuminating the dynamic workings of the mind. For this reason, it is often called *psychodynamic* psychotherapy. Another term for this type of therapy is *insight-oriented* psychotherapy, emphasizing the therapy's goal of helping the patient gain insights into the intricate dynamics underlying her thoughts and emotions. When used in patients who have borderline personality disorder, the goals and course are essentially the same—and can be effective—but progress can be slow and prolonged. Psychodynamic psychotherapy also requires thoughtful and objective introspection on the part of the patient, and though some persons who have BPD are ready to embark on such a process, most are not. The treatment of a person with repeated cutting behaviors, for example, needs to focus on these behaviors quickly and effectively. Also, if the patient's problems with behavior cause therapy sessions to continually focus on crises and dealing with emergencies, the patient won't have the time, let alone be in the thoughtful state of mind, required to develop new understandings. Although persons who have borderline personality disorder can and do benefit from psychodynamic psychotherapy, most need to initially focus on stopping behaviors rather than gaining insights—again, knowing why one engages in certain behaviors doesn't mean one will be able to stop them.

Several new therapies focused primarily on a patient's behaviors have been developed to meet these needs. These techniques turn the theory underlying psychodynamic therapy on its head in a sense, focusing on behavior first and assuming that the actions (that is, the behaviors) of a person are important causes of his emotional distress and problems in life. Therefore, if the behaviors are changed, the feelings and ways of thinking will naturally improve afterward. These therapies have certain advantages, particularly for people who have disorders that primarily involve what they *do*, for example, cutting behaviors, repeated suicidal behaviors, drug addiction and alcohol abuse, where understanding the problem does not necessarily change the behavior. In persons who have BPD, problematic behaviors are often a huge part of the problem, certainly the most disruptive for the individual and those around him, and are the source of much impairment in functioning. The benefits of psychodynamic therapy will be discussed in more detail in later chapters. Here we would like to focus on therapies specifically targeting maladaptive behaviors.

Cognitive Behavioral Therapy

Before the mid-twentieth century, the standard of care for most psychiatric disorders was psychoanalytic psychotherapy. This treatment method originally devised by Freud at the end of the nineteenth century has constantly evolved over the decades, occasionally splitting into additional schools, but always focusing on the unconscious processes of the mind. Psychoanalysts work to bring the patient's unconscious thoughts and motivations into the conscious mind and assume that when a person understands the unconscious forces at work behind his feelings and worldly interactions, he will be able to improve them.

During the 1950s, however, more and more therapists became frustrated with this form of therapy for many reasons. It required many years of (costly) training to master *after* becoming a psychiatrist or psychologist and was prohibitively expensive for all but a few patients. In addition, many patients did not find the therapy practical, because it required meeting with the analyst for four or five hours a week, often for many years, to make progress. Perhaps most important, a much greater awareness of how common psychological problems like depression are made it clear that more efficient treatment methods were urgently needed; at the same time, the work of professionals other than psychiatrists, such as clinical psychologists and social workers, was proving effective in mental health clinics. A flurry of new therapies started to appear, and they shared several common characteristics: most were short term (patients were in therapy for weeks or months rather than years), the patient and therapist usually met only once a week, and the therapist and the patient focused on relieving symptoms and solving problems rather than on understanding the unconscious. One of these, usually most associated with Dr. Aaron Beck at the University of Pennsylvania, has stood the test of time.

In the 1960s, dissatisfied with the psychoanalytic treatment of patients with depression, Dr. Beck came to the conclusion that addressing the manner in which his patients interacted with the world was the key to their problems. This included, most important, their perceptions of their environment and how they interpreted or thought about it. From these conclusions, he went on to create cognitive therapy, *cognitive* from the word *cognition*, the psychological term for "thinking." Dr. Beck came to believe that depressed persons had developed negative ways of thinking because of adverse experiences early in life, such that they focused on the negative aspects of their environment and tended to ignore the positive.

Over the next ten years, Beck gradually incorporated treatment approaches that were based on theories of psychology born nearly eighty years earlier in the animal laboratory of Ivan Pavlov. As its name suggests, *behavioral theory* (or *behavioralism*) focuses on what people *do*, and considers the mind a "black box" whose workings are essentially unknowable. Further developed by psychologist B. F. Skinner and others who applied the theory to humans in the 1950s, behavioralism proposes that what people do—and also what they think and feel, considering thinking and feeling as simply additional forms of behavior—is molded by the consequences of their behavior. If the person is rewarded by the environment for a certain behavior, he will tend to repeat it. If punished for a particular behavior, he is less likely to repeat it. Anyone who has trained his dog not to jump up on the furniture, or to sit when told, has, in a sense, been using the techniques of behavioral therapy.

Cognitive behavioral therapy (CBT) combines elements drawn from both theories and, like both of them, focuses on the here and now. It is based on the idea that negative feelings come from and are sustained by ingrained negative thinking patterns (the *cognitive* aspect of the theory), and that these thinking patterns can be challenged and changed so that more positive feelings and healthier ways of interacting in the world will result (the *behavioral* aspect).

CBT has additional advantages over other forms of therapy. For one thing, it can be highly standardized and has even been reduced to manuals for therapists that lay out the details of weekly sessions. These manuals contain a "lesson plan" for what is to occur in each session, and handouts, or "homework," for the patient to complete between sessions. The duration of CBT treatment is often much shorter than psychodynamic psychotherapy—in some studies, twelve weeks has been shown to produce a marked improvement in a given problem. These advantages made CBT available to more patients, who were more accepting of it, not only because the theory is easier to understand than many other types of therapy, but also because it focuses on problem behaviors and current functioning.

CBT: A Closer Look

In Aaron Beck's first book, published in 1967, called *Depression: Causes and Treatment,* he describes the cognitive aspects of the theory and treatment.[2] Beck believed that the central cause of low mood and depression was the tendency of a person to have negative thoughts about the world and herself, and that the person developed this pattern of thinking as a result of early negative interactions with the world (being put down by her peers, repeatedly disappointed by her parents, etc.). The cognitive theory of depression proposes that this pattern of thinking becomes a habit, so that any slightly negative stimulus the person encounters will set it off again.

A more traditional psychodynamic psychotherapist might address this pattern by having the patient recall her early negative experiences in detail and examine what exactly occurred during the experience and what feelings it set off, with the hope of eventually realizing how these past experiences and feelings are affecting her present. Beck took a different approach. He believed that *how* the pattern became established was not all that important—what was important was *changing* this thinking pattern in the here and now. This is done by challenging the individual's negative thoughts and cognitions, and training the person to have more positive thoughts, with the expectation that emotions will improve in turn.

Beck proposed several common patterns of negative thinking that he called *cognitive distortions*, which have the effect of making the person perceive the world in a relentlessly negative light and not as it actually is. For example, a person may tend to *catastrophize*. ("Because I missed this bus, I will be late for work, and my boss will probably see me come in late, then the project will never get done on time, and I'll be seen as lazy and probably get fired," rather than, "I'll just catch the next bus and hope for the best.") Another distortion is when a person mistakes her interpretation of certain facts for the facts themselves, and therefore sees no alternative viewpoints (thinking "Mike doesn't like me" instead of simply "Mike didn't wave at me in the hallway; perhaps he was preoccupied and didn't see me"). *Polarization* is a particularly common cognitive distortion among persons who have borderline personality disorder—tending to perceive others as either all good or all bad. If a friend picks you up from the airport, he is the most responsible, loving person ever! But if he is a few minutes late to meet for dinner the next day, he is uncaring, irresponsible, selfish, and not worth any attention.

Just about now, you may be wondering, "I thought this chapter was about changing *behaviors*; what's all this about *thoughts* and *feelings*?"

Here's the behavior part: the theory states that these false cognitions inevitably lead to negative behaviors of one type or another (the person who is late because he missed his bus will be nervous and distracted at work and not perform at his best), and the negative consequences that ensue (like the boss making a critical comment) not only have the effect of making the patient feel worse but also reinforce his depressive cognitive distortions ("I can't do anything right!"). As you can see, the negative thinking leads to negative behavior, which reinforces the negative thinking, and a vicious cycle ensues that makes it almost impossible to interrupt the behavior.

The first step in treatment is to educate the patient about what CBT is and how the theory works. The second step is to find out what problems he would like to work on. Then the patient is given homework, the first assignment often being to simply pay attention to and write down related cognitions (that is, thoughts), feelings, and behaviors in detail. One of Beck's premises is that these patterns (of thinking and behaving) are so ingrained that they are unconscious—the person is not even aware of them; for example, catastrophizing becomes so much a part of a person's daily life that he no longer realizes that it is happening. By writing down in detail the episodes that trouble the person, he begins to identify the connections between his negative actions and negative thoughts.

This homework is then brought to the next session and discussed with the therapist, who helps the patient connect the dots between negative thoughts and negative behaviors and work on replacing the distorted thinking patterns with more logical ones. The therapist does this by actively challenging the negative cognitions ("Would your boss *really* fire you for being late to work one day?") and asking the patient to come up with a more logical way of thinking about the episode ("No one gets fired for being late only once in a great while. There was really nothing to fret about"). After that, the therapist usually teaches the patient something new. This may be a new technique to deal with anxiety, such as progressive muscle relaxation, or positive alternative thinking patterns to replace the habitual negative ones (a technique called cognitive restructuring). At the end of the session, new homework is assigned. This process is repeated until the patient begins to make progress.

Another method that CBT uses to change behavior focuses on connecting negative behaviors to the negative thinking that is so automatic the person isn't even aware of the process (sometimes called *automatic thoughts*). This technique is called *exposure-response prevention* and is in many ways one of the cornerstones of cognitive behavioral therapy. The first goal of this technique is to help the person recognize the automatic ways in which she responds to stimuli (breaking up with her significant other because of one missed phone call, or threatening to kill herself after a fight). She is given homework to write down negative situations and how she responded to them (and, if possible, her cognitions as well, because this information is useful for different exercises). The patient then runs through a cost-benefit analysis of these particular coping mechanisms with the therapist and is helped to realize just how maladaptive they are. The next step is for the patient to estimate how hard it would be to refrain from these behaviors and rate them on a scale of easiest to prevent to hardest to prevent. The behaviors are then systematically dealt with, usually from easiest to hardest.

The patient is asked to identify what cognitions and feelings occur in the split second between the stimuli and the response. Often, she is surprised by the richness of emotion and cognition that occurs in this short period, as the experiences had been pretty much automatic. Cognitive exercises, which essentially consist of analyzing the distorted thinking and the behavior it triggers, can be used to help the patient develop a rationale as to why the behavior is a poor coping mechanism. She is then told that the next time she is exposed to the stimulus, she is to refrain from the behavior. This may provoke significant anxiety for the patient ("Can I do it?" "How will I do it?" "What if I fail—will my therapist leave me?"). The therapist will reassure her that these worries are natural, and together, therapist and patient explore how to address them, mainly by working on possible alternative behaviors. This is often the foundation of a homework assignment—the patient is told to draw up a list, a "safety plan," for what she will do *instead* of the negative behavior. At the next session, the list is reviewed with the therapist, and the patient may even mentally practice going down the list in the session.

The patient is then told to take the process one step further, to again identify some negative stimulus and her response to it, but this time, instead of simply writing down the stimulus-emotion/cognition-response cycle, she is told to *prevent* the automatic response, going down her list of alternative coping techniques as needed until she feels better, then writing down what she thinks and how she feels about the experience. When she has alternative coping mechanisms successfully in place to prevent one behavior and is relatively comfortable not responding in her typical, maladaptive way, another behavior is addressed, one further up the hierarchy of difficulty. This is repeated (with "touch ups" for previous behaviors as necessary) until all problem behaviors have been addressed.

The efficacy of CBT has been proven many times in research studies for various diagnoses. Specific programs have been developed for depression, anxiety, PTSD, obsessive-compulsive disorder, and other diagnoses. Several studies of the efficacy of CBT in persons who have borderline personality disorder show that it is effective at reducing self-harm and destructive behaviors.[3,4] In 2006, the first research study to compare the efficacy of CBT against other forms of psychotherapy for persons who have borderline personality disorder was published. The Borderline Personality Disorder Study of Cognitive Therapy (BOSCOT) trial was carried out at three clinics in England and Scotland and compared a group of patients who had borderline personality disorder and received "usual treatment" with another group who received CBT in addition to their usual treatment. The addition of CBT decreased the number of suicidal acts of patients and reduced anxiety and *dysfunctional beliefs* (distorted negative thinking patterns). However, there was no significant difference between the groups in the number of cutting and other self-mutilation episodes, nor in the number of emergency room visits or psychiatric hospitalizations. While somewhat encouraging, these results are nevertheless disappointing because of the lack of behavioral change. Also, it's important to note that the persons who received CBT plus treatment as usual received a higher "dose" of psychotherapy than the non-CBT group. Did the CBT group do somewhat better because of the CBT—or just because they had more therapeutic contact?

Perhaps these patients didn't have more improvement in self-harming behaviors because they weren't quite ready for standard CBT; perhaps they needed a form of CBT that is more specialized and specific to their problems. In the next section we will discuss just such a treatment.

Dialectical Behavioral Therapy

In 1987, Dr. Marsha Linehan, a psychology professor at the University of Washington, published a paper in which she outlined an adaptation of the principles of CBT developed specifically for the treatment of individuals who had borderline personality disorder.[5] Called *dialectical behavior therapy* (DBT), it has been the most widely studied form of psychotherapy for this diagnosis.

The word *dialectic* originated with the philosophers of ancient Greece and evolved in the works of other philosophers to include various ways of thinking about opposites. The German philosopher Georg Hegel believed that it was possible to consider opposite ideas in such a way as to realize that they are both part of a higher truth. The opposite ideas he designated by the terms *thesis* and *antithesis*. The process of combining them to comprehend something more fundamental he called *synthesis*. DBT considers several dialectics, perhaps the most important being the synthesis of the idea that the self-destructive behaviors of the person who has BPD represent her best efforts to cope and to feel and function better with a seemingly opposite idea: she needs to do better. The therapist and the patient work on continually finding a balance between acceptance and change, with the ultimate goal of eliminating dysfunctional coping strategies and replacing them with more effective strategies so that the patient can grow as a person and live a happier, more fulfilled life.

Linehan's emphasis on this dialectic can be understood as arising from her conceptualization of the causes of behavioral problems in individuals with BPD: the combination of internal (biological) and external (environmental) forces acting on a person's psyche—a way of thinking that will be familiar to you from our discussion of the four psychiatric perspectives.

The biological factors in persons who have BPD result in their intense *emotional reactivity*, which itself consists of three parts. First is extreme sensitivity to emotional stimuli. Even a small environmental stimulus, which may be overlooked by most people, can provoke a reaction. The second is emotional intensity—these emotional stimuli not only provoke a reaction, but an *extreme* or very strong reaction. The third part is a slowness to return to emotional baseline—this means that extreme reactions are prolonged, and it is difficult for the person to bring himself back down to stability. This description of the biological factors looks at the problems from the disease as well as the dimensional perspectives.

Regarding the environmental factors, Linehan proposes that these individuals have often spent much of their early life in environments she refers to as "invalidating." Because important people in the person's life don't understand the intensity and reactivity of her emotions, they often discount (invalidate) the person's distress by saying something like "Stop crying, you can't possibly be *that* upset!" Or perhaps they try to soothe the upset youngster for a time but then give up and ignore her. Linehan reports that her own patients have often experienced far more than their share of unfair criticism from family members, who have labeled the child's emotional distress as lack of discipline, immaturity, or just not trying hard enough. When important persons in the environment repeatedly label a child's angry feelings as "just being hateful," or say to the tearful child "you're not sad; you're just acting like a baby," the child doesn't learn to comprehend her private experiences. The disconnect between the emotional turmoil inside and how others are reacting to her (ignoring or discounting her emotions) and what they are saying to her ("Just stop it; there's nothing to be upset about") makes it difficult for the child to label emotions accurately, to appropriately communicate how she is feeling to others, and, most important, to understand the causes of uncomfortable feelings and means of controlling them. These problems in turn interfere with the process of learning the typical give-and-take of interpersonal relationships, not to mention grasping how one's emotional reactions affect others.

What *do* tend to get reinforced are ever more intense emotional displays, which can be understood as the individual's attempt to get some control over this unpredictable environment. As Dr. Linehan has put it, "Within an invalidating environment, extreme emotional displays and/ or extreme problems are often necessary to provoke a helpful environment."[6] But these extremes lead to even more negative reactions from the environment, often because the intensity of the emotional displays seems unpredictable and inconsistent—and therefore willful—even to the most patient caretaker, and the cycle continues. The behaviors, cognitions, and emotions that are clustered together under the name of borderline personality disorder are increasingly entrenched, a process that will be familiar from our earlier discussion of behavioral theory. Because the person doesn't have the communication skills to express emotions accurately or the problem-solving skills necessary for effectively dealing with whatever precipitated the emotional crisis, she can only express emotional distress with escalating behaviors in an effort to be seen and taken seriously by those around her.

In standard cognitive behavioral therapy (CBT), the goal of the treatment is to change the person in a positive direction. But if the person has borderline personality disorder, this constant push to change can easily be interpreted by him as just another invalidating, unsupportive, and confrontational environment. This can lead to him withdrawing from or terminating treatment or becoming agitated and aggressive. This is where the dialectical stance comes in: remember that *dialectical* refers to the idea of holding two different goals and assumptions in mind simultaneously. The DBT therapist works on synthesizing the process of validating the patient's feelings and actions as they are right now, in any given moment, but at the same time demanding that the patient change. Confrontation must be perfectly balanced with acceptance.

In fact, these "dialectical dilemmas," as Linehan calls them, are also useful in thinking about the seemingly distorted thinking and perplexing behaviors of the person with BPD. For example, consider a person with the borderline diagnosis who frequently makes suicidal statements. Such individuals often *simultaneously* want to live and want to die. Saying aloud to another person, "I want to die" (rather than killing oneself in secrecy) shows some indication that the person also wants to live. However, for the therapist to make that observation (for example, "You wouldn't have told me that if you *really* wanted to die") would be to invalidate that patient's desire not to live his life *as it currently is*. It is not true that the low lethality of a suicidal statement means that the person does not *really* want to die. It is not necessarily even that the person alternates between the two—the individual simultaneously holds both opposing desires and beliefs in his mind *at the same time*.

Those close to individuals with a borderline diagnosis are often familiar with the experience of being loved absolutely one minute and hated absolutely the next. This black-and-white thinking is characteristic of these individuals, who have difficulty finding any gray zone in situations or people. The title of a book for therapists about treating these patients, *I Hate You, Don't Leave Me,* aptly captures the idea. One of the goals of DBT is to teach persons who have borderline personality disorder how to find the gray zones between emotional extremes, and one of the core tenets of DBT is to constantly strive for this gray, sometimes called the "middle path." (If this reminds you of Zen philosophy, it should. Zen principles have also informed the development of DBT.)

DBT is structured according to five separate domains of treatment, each with its own setting and cast of characters. The first of these is *capability enhancement,* which focuses on improved behavioral and emotional self-regulation. This usually takes place in meetings in which the therapist instructs a group of patients in coping skills and techniques. (These groups are not like standard group therapy, where a therapist facilitates patients' sharing of their feelings and experiences; rather, the structure for the meetings is more like a classroom, with the therapist as instructor and the patients in the roles of learners.) The patients are instructed in different skills, including mindfulness (another Zen principle), improving control of attention and the mind by focusing on the here and now to reduce emotional intensity, enhancing interpersonal skills and conflict management, and increasing their ability to tolerate distress. This focus on teaching skills for self-improvement is the facet of DBT that most closely mirrors CBT. Linehan saw this step as essential, but not sufficient, for the treatment of borderline personality disorder.

The second domain is *motivation enhancement*. As opposed to skill teaching, this must be performed in individual (one-on-one) therapy sessions. In this facet of treatment, the therapist ensures that progress is reinforced and that maladaptive behavior is not. Often, the therapist asks the patient to track problem behaviors and thinking patterns in a diary. False beliefs and cognitions are challenged, but (of course) this is always balanced with empathic validation of the patient as she is right now. The essence of validation consists of listening empathetically, reflecting accurately, articulating what is experienced but not necessarily said, clarifying which of the patient's behaviors are disordered, and highlighting those behaviors that are valid because they fit current facts or are effective for the patient's long-term goals. In a process called *behavioral chain analysis*, therapist and patient explore everything that led up to, occurred during, and resulted from an incident of problem behavior and try to identify options for more skillful and effective responses. Most important, the therapist must be seen by the patient, and respond to the patient, as a person of equal status and value. The relationship that develops is critical for the progress of the therapy.

The third domain is *enhancing generalization*. Lessons learned during capability and motivation enhancement are useless unless they can be taken outside the therapist's office and generalized to the external environment. This domain takes place on an "as needed" basis, usually over the phone. For example, the patient who experiences a stressful event or overwhelming emotion in the real world is instructed to contact her therapist instead of responding in her usual maladaptive way. The therapist's role is to encourage the patient to de-escalate the situation and her emotions using the skills the patient has learned up to this point. This step in the treatment serves many different functions. It supports the patient in her time of worry and reinforces the bond between patient and therapist. At the same time, it seeks to avoid the patient's developing dependence on other people by encouraging her to use the skills they have been working on in individual and group sessions, thus fostering independence and self-reliance. The patient may be coached over the phone on using her skills to de-escalate the situation (for example putting into action a previously developed emergency plan that can include calling 911 or going to an emergency room). This strategy reinforces the role of the therapist as a supportive figure in the patient's life, but strives to help the person break from maladaptive behavioral patterns by forcing her to take responsibility for her own actions, and not allowing the therapist to be manipulated into flying immediately to the patient's rescue.

Our discussion has focused on supporting the patient, but this form of treatment can be quite stressful for the therapist. This is why the fourth domain of treatment, *therapist consultation,* consists of maintaining the motivation and capabilities of the therapist. People who have borderline personality disorder commonly escalate situations around them to incite crises capable of evoking strong emotions in other people—including their therapist. Built into DBT is a regular "supervision," or support group meeting for DBT therapists, usually weekly, to discuss their own strong emotional reactions to patients' manipulative behaviors and how to best handle them. It serves not only as a way to plan treatment strategies, but also to ensure that the treatment is not derailed by the therapists' own negative reactions to their patients.

The fifth and final domain of treatment consists of *structuring the environment.* Remember that borderline behavior in now usually conceptualized as a complex interaction of the person's own biological endowment and a negative, invalidating environment. It is therefore impossible to treat the patient in isolation without also addressing his negatively reinforcing surroundings. This is extremely important if gains made in treatment are to persist after terminating therapy. The therapist will work hard to coach the patient on how to communicate more effectively with family members and others in the environment, but if necessary, family meetings involving the important people in the patient's life may be built into the structure of DBT to discuss treatment strategies and ongoing interpersonal conflict. This window into the patient's environment can allow the therapist to target specific areas of difficulty. Sometimes the therapist will note that families have their own negative reactions to the patient and will set up an emergency plan similar to the "enhancing generalization" plan above, incorporating familial support while fostering the patient's independence and self-reliance. At other times, the therapist may note that the other members of the patient's social circle have their own unique problems that require individual attention and can make therapeutic referrals on their behalf.

The foregoing discussion of DBT actually describes only its first phase. In the second phase, the DBT therapist begins to help the patient better understand and make peace with the early life experiences that contributed to her difficulties. This is not so different from more traditional psychodynamic therapy, which we will discuss below and in the next chapter. After helping the patient deal with the past, DBT enters a third and then a fourth phase, in which treatment focuses on improving the patient's quality of life and the ability to experience joy.

THE EFFECTIVENESS OF DBT for persons who have borderline personality disorder has been demonstrated in many clinical studies. In the first of these, forty-seven chronically suicidal BPD patients at the University of Washington were randomly assigned for a year either to DBT or to treatment as usual in the community. During the year, DBT patients were less likely to attempt suicide or drop out (84 percent remained in treatment). They spent much less time in psychiatric hospitals, had greater reductions in use of psychotropic medications, and were better adjusted at the end of the year. They were also less angry than patients given standard psychotherapy (although at one year, they were not less depressed or less likely to think about suicide). Most of these differences persisted a year after treatment ended.[7] DBT has also proven effective in reducing substance abuse among persons who have BPD. Twenty-three drug-abusing women who had borderline personality disorder were assigned to DBT or to treatment as usual in the community. At the end of the one-year treatment, use of illicit drugs was lower and attendance at treatment was higher in the patients who got DBT versus those referred to treatment as usual.[8]

A criticism of these studies is that they have been carried out by a team of researchers headed by the person who developed DBT, Dr. Linehan. However, these are early days in the development of psychotherapeutic techniques specifically for the condition, so this should not be too surprising. The developers of any new treatment intervention frequently dominate the research literature on the technique initially, with independent studies to follow that replicate (or refute) the earlier studies.

DBT'S FOCUS on the dialectical dilemmas that people who have BPD face daily, and on the therapist's addressing them from a nonjudgmental standpoint, may be why it is generally liked and well tolerated by persons who have borderline personality disorder. The treatment is quite intensive during some of its phases, but this is a necessary part of a treatment plan with such extensive built-in support for both the patient and the therapist. Not only does it address the distress and disordered behavior of the individual, but it also pays special attention to addressing the person's surroundings (family and environment) and the stresses and emotional reactivity of the therapist. By meeting in weekly support sessions, and teaching the patient particular protocols to follow if he begins to feel suicidal, DBT places a strict frame around the relationship between the therapist and the patient that makes them both feel safe and more comfortable.

CHAPTER 11

Understanding the Dimensions and Addressing the Life Story

MAGGIE WAS TAKING A YEAR OFF *before starting college. She was intelligent and charming, had been a good student in high school, and by all accounts was headed for a successful life. However, when her boyfriend Tom left to attend university in another town, many things about Maggie changed.*

Maggie and Tom had made an agreement to talk by phone once a day after dinner. At first, this went well, but then Maggie began texting Tom throughout the day as well. He soon found that if he was even a few minutes "late" answering the after-dinner call with her, Maggie would quickly become upset, convinced that he was having a good time without her and was losing interest in their relationship. The same thing started to happen if Tom did not reply to her text messages immediately. One evening, the charge on Tom's phone had run out without him realizing it, and the next thing he knew Maggie was knocking at the door of his dorm room—she had driven three hours to the university to confront him, very upset, convinced that he was cheating on her. It took hours to calm her down, and she was so distraught that he insisted she stay the night with him.

The next day, though, it seemed as if she had forgotten the whole thing had happened. "Since I'm already here, I'll stay till Monday and we can be together all weekend!" Tom had other plans, but he worried about how Maggie would react to this, so he sent a few texts on the sly to cancel them.

As Maggie was driving home Monday morning, she started thinking about all the other women she had seen on campus, and started worrying again that Tom wasn't in love with her.

The next Friday night, she called Tom on the way home from a party,

174

but he didn't pick up. She left a message that she was going home "to spend the night with a bottle of Tylenol" because "without you, what's the point of living?" Things got much worse after that.

Maggie had been progressing fairly well with her new DBT group work and individual therapy. She hadn't cut herself in months. The urges were still there, but she had found other ways to deal with them.

She still thought about taking an overdose—a lot—but she'd started to understand that it wouldn't solve her problems. She had even thrown away the stash of pills she had kept in her closet "in case life got to be too much." The end of her most recent relationship four months ago had been the trigger for her last suicide attempt, and she had successfully avoided getting into another romantic relationship by spending more time with her family.

But, she was frustrated—she had made so many changes in her life, why couldn't anyone else see it? Mom and Dad were still distant with her at times (which really triggered her urges to cut), she was still having trouble with her friends . . . what was their deal? Didn't they trust that she was better? It just made her so angry sometimes. "I'll never get better in this terrible environment!" And her family was setting her up to fail—of course she was going to get mad at them if they didn't invite her to see that movie (although she'd relentlessly made fun of them for wanting to see such a stupid movie in the first place). She'd earned that right! Maybe they wanted her to fail, to kill herself; that way they wouldn't have to deal with her.

In this situation, Maggie was indeed progressing in her treatment; her problems with "borderline behaviors" had greatly improved. She still had some negative thinking patterns: when her family didn't invite her to see a movie that she had said she didn't want to see, she took it as a personal assault. But Maggie is not adept at patience. She takes for granted that the progress she has made and her intentions to continue getting better should automatically be accepted by everyone around her—and that they should just forget the past: the crazy phone calls, the tantrums, the suicide attempts. She does not yet understand the deep rifts her behaviors have torn in these relationships, and how long it will take for these to heal. Furthermore, at times, she still feels so bad about herself and becomes so overemotional that she has urges to cut. She has successfully dealt with the *behavior* of cutting, she knows how to interrupt it now, but she has not yet addressed the feelings behind this behavior.

When persons who have the BPD diagnosis are progressing along well in changing their behaviors, how can they address the sort of emotional dross that is left over? How do they bring some insight into emotional states and expectations in a way that reduces their internal distress (as much as the behavioral therapies reduce the distress they may give to others)? The family of psychodynamic psychotherapies fills just such a role in treatment.

Using our formulation of the causes and factors that result in the multifaceted set of problems called borderline personality disorder, we have now reached the point where we will survey the treatments that focus on *who the person is*, that aim to actually change personality by helping the individual smooth the sharp edges of his extremes of temperament that contribute to his difficulties. A related goal is to help the person make sense out of *what he has encountered*, and to realize how his emotional reactions in the present are sometimes rooted in past experiences that can still have the power to drive his emotional life.

In the late nineteenth century, Sigmund Freud revolutionized the understanding and treatment of mental illness when he developed a sophisticated system of illuminating human behavior based on understanding childhood development. He and his followers developed a "talking treatment" for psychiatric problems: psychotherapy. This basically consists of helping patients get to know themselves better, so that based on this knowledge, they can let go of their grudges, resentments, and fears that are rooted in past experiences and learn better, more mature ways of understanding themselves and others, as well as more effective coping mechanisms. The approach is called *psychodynamic psychotherapy* and is based on the belief that mental life is best understood as a dynamic interplay between emotions and intellect, present circumstances and unconscious memories of past experiences, and many other psychological factors.

Psychodynamic psychotherapy's focus on a person's past emotions and experiences is based on the assumption that only by exploring and grasping the interplay of emotions and experiences in the past, and how these have helped create the present situation, can a person change her present situation; only after identifying the negative patterns of thinking, acting, and reacting in a person's life can she stop repeating them. Psychodynamic therapy differs from CBT and the initial phase of DBT in the way it emphasizes emotions and experiences rather than behaviors, as well as past and present interpersonal relationships (including the therapeutic relationship) and the interpretation of the patient's wishes, dreams, and fantasies.[1] Behavioral therapies (like CBT and DBT's initial phase) focus almost exclusively on the present and largely ignore the past. Behavioral approaches focus on how to deal with things *now* and set up protocols and coping mechanisms to function in the *future*. But the past is considered almost irrelevant.

Until the 1990s, psychodynamic therapies were the primary psychotherapeutic technique for persons with the BPD diagnosis. With the development of behavioral treatments that are effective in helping persons interrupt the distressing and disturbing behaviors of borderline personality disorder, psychodynamic psychotherapy fell out of favor for a time. This is largely because many practitioners had treated patients who were willing to discuss their emotional world and past experiences but were still not able to make many real changes in their present or future *behaviors*. This ineffectiveness for many of these people led to the switch in focus to the more present-based, problem-solving behavioral therapies like CBT and DBT.

More recently, practitioners have begun to take a second look at whether psychodynamic psychotherapies can be helpful and how they can be incorporated into the treatment of borderline personality disorder. There are currently two schools of thought on what the role for psychodynamic psychotherapy in treating borderline personality disorder should be.

The first of these is that psychodynamic psychotherapy should be complementary to a behavioral therapy; many clinicians offer psychodynamic psychotherapy only *after* the patient has made significant progress in extinguishing self-destructive behaviors and has become much more adept at managing feelings. Only after DBT's first phase has helped the patient learn techniques for stopping self-destructive behaviors will he have the emotional resilience to start phase two to work on recognizing and coming to terms with who he is, and with the accumulated consequences of a lifetime of tense interpersonal relationships caused by these behaviors. Past traumatic experiences that have contributed to a person's troubles are also addressed using this form of therapy.

There are several reasons for this plan of sequenced psychotherapy, that is, focusing on stopping problem behaviors at the beginning of treatment followed by psychodynamic psychotherapy. One is that a person who is still buffeted by unmanageable emotions simply can't manage the calm self-reflection that is crucial for successful psychodynamic psychotherapy. Another is that the person who is still not in control of self-destructive behaviors and is still lurching from crisis to crisis will have neither the time nor the emotional resources needed to address long-term problems. Crisis management will inevitably become all-consuming of therapy resources; this is fine, of course, for DBT, which was designed specifically to help the patient learn crisis-management techniques, but psychodynamic psychotherapy requires a focus and continuity of process that repeated interruptions to manage crises will simply demolish. Perhaps most important, psychotherapy almost inevitably stirs up anxiety and strong emotions as the person recalls and processes the past. This is especially true if the individual has been a victim of trauma. Unless the individual has the coping mechanisms to deal with these emotions, psychotherapy will result in worsened symptoms rather than improvement.

The idea is that the more reflective, introspective approach of psychodynamic psychotherapy helps the person who has already learned to control behaviors and to cope with extreme emotions to embark on the process of understanding himself in a more profound way that isn't just focused on getting rid of symptoms but that leads to real personal growth and the process of becoming a happier, more fulfilled person.

For this purpose, psychodynamic psychotherapy as it has long been practiced is the best method. Since the person's self-destructive behaviors and problems with continual crises have stopped, he will benefit from the same approach that is used for anyone having difficulties such as making good decisions or solving problems with relationships. Perhaps a therapist who is a bit more patient and skilled is required for him at this point, but a psychodynamic approach specific to persons with the borderline diagnosis is not required. Sessions are usually once a week, for a period of many months, perhaps several years.

Psychodynamic Therapies for Borderline Personality Disorder

Contrasting with the idea that psychodynamic therapy is a useful *addition* to behavioral therapies is the theoretical stance that the patient must *always* find and understand the reasons behind his behaviors to end them, and that psychodynamic psychotherapy is therefore more effective than behaviorally oriented treatments like DBT and schema-based treatment. This idea also assumes that understanding and insight will automatically lead to behavioral changes and that techniques like DBT are simply not necessary. In the remainder of this chapter, we discuss three types of psychodynamic psychotherapy that have been developed specifically for the treatment of borderline personality disorder, and for which there is research evidence for efficacy. These approaches were developed because of the recognition that psychodynamic psychotherapy as it was practiced in the past was not effective for persons who had BPD and the realization that psychodynamic therapy would not be successful unless modified to specifically address the problems of these individuals.

We want to warn you at this point that the rest of this chapter may be tough going for many readers. Psychodynamic theory is highly complex, less than intuitive, abstract, and quite difficult to grasp initially. However, following through on our promise not to oversimplify, we review the theoretical underpinnings of several forms of psychotherapy developed specifically for the treatment of borderline personality disorder in a fair amount of detail. This may be of only limited interest to patients and their friends and family members; if you want to skip the rest of this chapter, no one will be insulted. You can move on to the next without any loss of continuity.

ONE OF THE BIGGEST COMPLEXITIES of psychodynamic therapy is that there are nearly as many forms of psychotherapy as practitioners, because each person does therapy in a slightly different and personal way. We know from research on psychodynamic psychotherapy that its success or failure is often more related to the personal qualities and experience of the therapist than the details of her techniques. To address this problem and increase the likelihood of successful therapy for all patients, attempts have been made to better standardize psychodynamic therapy, the way CBT and DBT are standardized. This standardization involves training therapists in the details of their practice techniques by using a kind of technical training manual: these techniques are then said to be *manualized.*

A happy consequence of creating a manual for psychotherapy is that it makes controlled research on specific types of therapy possible. More and more forms of psychodynamic therapy are being regimented and manualized in this way—both to increase their clinical usefulness and to make it possible to scientifically assess their efficacy.

Two forms of specialized psychodynamic therapy have been developed and studied for the treatment of borderline personality disorder: *transference-focused psychotherapy* and *mentalization-based treatment.*

Transference-Focused Psychotherapy

Dr. Otto Kernberg of the Weill Cornell Medical Center in New York has been widely regarded as the leader in psychodynamic psychotherapy for the treatment of persons who have borderline personality disorder. He started writing theoretical papers and accounts of his successes with his patients in the 1970s and then worked to standardize his approaches to better research their effectiveness and to teach them to other clinicians. Kernberg and his colleagues eventually developed a manualized version of his techniques, which they called transference-focused psychotherapy (TFP). First published in 1989, this manual opened up a different approach to treating borderline personality disorder for therapists who had prior psychodynamic training and were more comfortable with this way of thinking.

Kernberg's theory of psychology is subtle and intricate and is derived from a school of Freudian thought called *object relations*. It proposes that each of us relates to the outside world by way of *internal* representations of our environment, especially internal representations of the important people in our lives. These representations consist of a memory of interacting with another person and the feelings associated with that interaction. For example, based on positive interactions with his mother, a young child will develop an internalized representation (or "object") of his mother that is associated with feelings of safety and nurturing (the "good mother"). But mothers must discipline misbehaving children occasionally as well, and object relations theory proposes that this leads the young child to develop an *additional* internal representation of his mother as mean and punishing, associated with feelings of fear or anger (the "bad mother").

When mom behaves in a way the child perceives as "mean," he instantly erupts with fear and hostility to the "bad mother," because the "good mother" is nowhere to be found. These two "objects" exist separately in the child's mind. As the child matures emotionally, he can appreciate that his mother may be a little short at times, especially if she's tired or stressed, but that she loves him all the same, and if he's a little patient and understanding, and perhaps soothes her a bit, everything will be fine. The two "mother objects" have combined to form more complex and accurate representation. Instead of "good mother" and "bad mother," there is only "mother"—sometimes nurturing and sometimes mean, but the same person. The feelings associated with mother become more nuanced as well, and a richer representation of this person develops. In the young child, this ambiguity is too frightening to acknowledge, the idea that "good mother" has a bad side is just too anxiety provoking, so the child refuses to see any "bad" in "good mother." The "mother objects" remain separate until the child is psychologically mature enough to tolerate the anxiety of this ambiguity.

Object relations theory also proposes that we develop internalized representation of ourselves as well, and that initially there are separate "self objects" such as a "good me," who deserves to be rewarded for good behavior, and the "naughty me," who deserves to be punished. The theory proposes that the relations between these objects also changes over time as the child matures, hence the name of the theory, *object relations.*

Kernberg proposed that in persons who have borderline personality disorder, largely because of problems with inconsistent or traumatic parenting, these early representations, or objects, do not combine as they should, leading to a fundamental disconnect in which the person can only see others as either all good or all bad but cannot incorporate both sets of associated feelings when relating to others. The theory proposes that this *splitting* causes persons who have borderline personality disorder to love someone one minute and despise them the next—to them, in some real sense, there are two different people. These problems with object representation affect what has been called the person's *self-structure* as well, preventing him from ever forming a clear and coherent sense of his own identity in terms of who he is, a problem Kernberg has called *identity diffusion.* The person's sense of himself and of others is polarized and unstable, and this unpredictability is a cause of profound distress.

This is (believe it or not) a *very* simplified description of object relations theory and leaves out an enormous amount of further details. The essential idea proposed by Kernberg is that the distorted thinking patterns, problems with relationships, and self-destructive behaviors of individuals who have BPD can all be understood as emerging from disturbed object relations.

TFP attempts to directly confront and resolve the syndrome of identity diffusion, primarily by promoting integration of object representations into more cohesive whole representations of the self and of others. With TFP, instead of seeing people (and, at times, himself) as all good or all bad, the person endeavors to see the complexity inherent in every individual and how this complexity can lead to more predictability and a better way to interact with the world. The therapist helps the patient identify and confront the way he sees only all good and all bad in his interactions and experiences with others. The initial focus for therapy sessions is usually on interactions between the therapist and the patient during treatment rather than analyzing past experiences.

Transference is the Freudian term for the perceptions and feelings the patient develops for his therapist during treatment, feelings that are distorted by his past experiences rather than based on real interactions, hence the term for this treatment, *transference focused.*

Telling the therapist that she is a horrible person and should go jump in a lake, or telling the therapist that he is sorry and what could he have been thinking, or even telling the therapist that he's in love with her are all seen as the patient's unhealthy attempts to control the therapy and avoid the anxiety engendered by personality change. The therapist works hard to interpret these statements and feelings rather than react to them.

TFP sessions are scheduled twice a week, and the average time spent in therapy is between one and four years. While this may seem like a long time, it is still considerably shorter than would be typical of traditional Freudian psychoanalysis.

What about crisis management? This is considered an intrusion into treatment that must be managed quickly, definitively, and with minimal drama. At the beginning of treatment, the consequences for behaviors such as cutting, drug use, and suicide attempts are clearly defined. They may include hospitalization and even treatment termination. Kernberg proposes that the strength of the therapeutic relationship and the patient's unwillingness to lose this essential support will allow him to self-regulate his emotions to such an extent that these behaviors will be extinguished altogether.

Therapist supervision is critical to the therapy and, as with DBT, is built into it. Providing therapists with peer support allows them to explore their own negative feelings about their patients in a productive way and can help them refocus the therapy if they begin to stray.

As you might gather from our description of object relations theory (and remember, we gave you a simplified version), it is an approach that requires advanced knowledge of and experience with psychoanalytic concepts and techniques, which require prolonged training to master and a significant amount of experience to do well. As such, it may be the most difficult form of psychotherapy specific to borderline personality disorder to learn and use comfortably—in most studies, already seasoned therapists had to study for a full year to attain correct adherence to the manual and competence in the techniques. Also, because self-destructive behaviors are not addressed directly, a patient whose therapy is frequently interrupted because of his inability to manage crises may have difficulty making progress.

There is only one controlled research trial of TFP to date; it showed TFP was as successful in reducing suicidal behaviors, anger, and impulsivity as DBT, and appeared to be superior to DBT in reducing assaultive behaviors.

Mentalization-Based Treatment

Mentalization is the ability to look inward at one's own mental processes as well as the ability to understand the states of mind of others. It is another form of psychodynamic psychotherapy that has been manualized and researched as to efficacy. The official manual for mentalization-based treatment (MBT) was not published until 2004, but early forms of this treatment were being used in the 1980s.

Developed by Peter Fonagy, a clinical psychologist and psychoanalyst at University College London, MBT proposes that the fundamental psychological problem faced by persons who have borderline personality disorder, the "broken part" that leads to their many dysfunctions, is in effect their "inner eye." While people usually learn some form or other of mentalization as an infant and in childhood as part of their maturational process, these individuals haven't. While young, the child becomes emotionally attached to her primary caregivers, usually her parents, and this attachment, as well as the time spent with them, gives her the opportunity to share experiences with them, experiences that are accompanied by emotional reactions: both the child's reactions and the caregiver's. Often, a child will see her own emotional reaction mirrored in her caregiver, an experience that can teach a child many things, such as:

- This other person outside me has feelings too. My feelings aren't the only ones that matter.
- This other person and I are having the same emotional reaction to the same circumstances, so emotional reactions can be predicted in others.
- This shared reaction represents a bond between us, so I am not alone.

When there is a failure in this process—because the caregiver does not accurately reflect the emotional reactions of the child, because the child doesn't trust the relationship with her caregiver (as in abused children), or because her own emotional states are so variable that her emotional reactions often don't match up with those around her—then her ability to "mentalize" fails to develop normally. Because she never really learns to reflect on her mental states or those of others, her own emotional reactions just seem to happen randomly, and the idea that other people have feelings that can be hurt is simply incomprehensible. At the other extreme, the person may try to deal with this unpredictability by ignoring her own emotions or even inappropriately projecting her own emotional state or intentions onto the other.

The therapeutic approach of mentalization-based therapy is significantly different from that used in TFP. The basic goal is for the patient to learn to mentalize, that is, to learn to think about and recognize, her own and others' mental states. As in TFP and unlike traditional psychodynamic therapy, the therapist intensely focuses on the current mental state of the patient in the here and now, avoiding explorations of past experiences and interpretations of past mental states. Unlike TFP, however, the goal of therapy is not for the patient to develop insight or realizations of how past experiences and patterns color the present, but rather to learn to "mentalize" going forward. The approach brings the patient's mental state "into the room" so that it can be examined and discussed, both by the patient and by the therapist. The focus is kept solely on what the patient is currently feeling during the experience and on the immediate predecessors to the emotional response so that the patient can consciously, actively track the cause-and-effect trail in her mental state changes.

MBT thus shares with DBT a focus on developing the ability to carefully analyze one's thinking processes. It does not, however, share DBT's focus on learning to manage behaviors. DBT teaches patients not only to recognize their inner distress, but also to accept and tolerate it— another difference between *mentalization* and the similarly sounding *mindfulness* approach of DBT. While DBT does not necessarily focus on the causes for emotional reactions, mentalization attempts to alleviate the internal conflicts that cause distress by giving patients the tools to look at themselves and others objectively rather than emotionally.

Mentalization-based treatment has been better studied than TFP. It was originally developed to be a day hospital–based treatment for patients from a relatively impoverished area in London who had borderline personality disorder. Here it was shown to be superior to traditional psychodynamic psychotherapy in reduced self-mutilation and suicidal acts, fewer days in the hospital, less use of psychotropic medications, improvement in anxiety and depressive symptoms, and better psychosocial functioning.

Schema-Focused Therapy

Some experts in the psychotherapeutic treatment of borderline personality disorder would object to our decision to review *schema-focused therapy* (SFT, or ST) in this chapter rather than in the previous chapter on behaviorally oriented treatments. This is because ST is an active therapeutic approach that focuses on identifying distorted thinking patterns and interrupting behaviors as cognitive behavioral therapy (CBT) and dialectical behavioral therapy (DBT) do. But like TFP, it is rooted in object relations theory and emphasizes the exploration of childhood experiences in the context of a supportive therapeutic relationship. ST has been developed largely by Dr. Jeffrey Young, a psychologist who worked with Aaron Beck, the originator of CBT.

As with the other treatments for persons with this diagnosis, SFT assumes that borderline personality disorder is caused by an interac-

Table II.I Examples of maladaptive schemas

Abandonment/instability: Persons available to the individual for support and connection are perceived as unstable or unreliable. This schema involves the sense that significant others will not be able to continue providing emotional support, connection, strength, or practical protection because they are emotionally unstable and unpredictable (e.g., have angry outbursts), unreliable, or present only erratically; because they will die imminently; or because they will abandon the individual in favor of someone better.

Mistrust/abuse: Others are expected to hurt, abuse, humiliate, cheat, lie, manipulate, or take advantage. This schema usually involves the perception that the harm is intentional or the result of unjustified and extreme negligence and may include the sense that one always ends up being cheated, or "getting the short end of the stick."

Emotional deprivation: This schema involves the expectation that one's desire for a normal degree of emotional support will not be adequately met by others.

Source: Adapted from J. Young et al., *Schema Therapy: A Practitioner's Guide* (New York: Guilford Press, 2003).

tion of genetic and temperamental factors with difficulties in early relationships, especially the child's relationships with her parents. These difficulties may be as traumatic as physical or sexual abuse or as subtle as a mismatch between the child's temperament and her parents' rearing style. The family environment is perceived as unsafe, depriving, rejecting, or frankly punitive (a similar idea to that of the "invalidating environment" that has been proposed by Marsha Linehan).

As a result of these negative childhood experiences, individuals who have BPD develop a variety of maladaptive schemas. The term *schema* is used in much the same way as in CBT, and maladaptive schemas are self-defeating emotional and thinking patterns that result in maladaptive behaviors (see table 11.1 for examples of maladaptive schemas).

Young also borrows from object relations theory and proposes that persons who have borderline personality disorder also have poorly integrated aspects of themselves that interact in destructive ways. These aspects of the person's identity are also likened to particular ways of behaving, grouped in constellations called *modes*. Modes can be triggered by the environment and lead to behaviors that characterize that mode. For example, a person who has BPD may "flip" (Young's term) into "Angry and Impulsive Child" mode when she perceives that her needs are not being met and erupt in rage.

The SFT therapist works to provide a supportive and predictably safe emotional environment (engaging the "Abandoned Child" mode) and to help the patient recognize and change her dysfunctional schemas and modes of reacting. Schema therapists also borrow behavioral and cognitive techniques from DBT and CBT that focus on daily life outside therapy as well as past experiences (including traumatic experiences). The patient recovers as her dysfunctional schemas no longer control her life.

Researchers in Holland compared the efficacy of SFT with TFP at four community mental health centers.[2] Patients saw a therapist twice a week for up to three years (a shorter period if they achieved recovery). Clinically significant improvements were found in both treatment groups on outcomes such as borderline symptoms and quality of life, but with greater improvement in the patient getting SFT. In addition, SFT led to significantly greater reduction in severity of nine of the DSM-IV criteria for BPD: identity disturbance, dissociation / paranoia, physically self-destructive acts and other forms of impulsivity, abandonment fears, and stormy relationships. Also, a greater percentage of SFT patients recovered, and fewer dropped out of treatment.

Psychotherapy for Borderline Personality Disorder: Summing Up

There are now quite a few studies on four forms of psychotherapy that have been especially developed to treat borderline personality disorder. For the purpose of this section, we will add dialectical behavioral therapy (DBT) to the discussion; although it is technically not a psychodynamic approach, it is psychotherapy and was developed especially for treating those who have BPD.

Although every one of these treatments is in the early days, the results of studies on their efficacy are quite encouraging. As one expert said in a paper reviewing comparison studies, "It is a real advance in the field that both clinicians and patients now have [several] treatments from which to choose. This is important as one treatment approach may make more sense to a particular clinician or a particular patient than the others."[3]

At this point, however, there is simply not enough research evidence to recommend one of these approaches over the others because few studies have compared one form of treatment with another. No research provides guidance regarding matching a particular approach to a particular patient. This means that clinicians must rely on their experience, skill, and that elusive quality called clinical wisdom to make these decisions. Choosing among several different effective treatments is a new problem for persons who have borderline personality disorder and for the clinicians charged with developing treatment plans for them—and frankly, it's a nice problem to have.

Of the four psychotherapy treatments that we have discussed, dialectical behavioral therapy has been the best studied and is also the most widely practiced. Will other approaches catch up as far as proven effectiveness and wider availability? Only time will tell. But after a period of doldrums in research on and development of new therapies for this disorder, we are now in a time of active research. These treatments will undoubtedly continue to be refined and perhaps more developed in coming years, and more research data will become available to assist patients and their clinicians in choosing a treatment with the best chance of success.

CHAPTER 12

Treatment Approaches

Putting It All Together

We have spent many pages attempting to unpack the complexity of borderline personality disorder. The framework that we have used to do this was developed at Johns Hopkins over several decades and proposes that understanding people who have any psychiatric problem requires viewing their difficulties from four different psychiatric perspectives.

The first of these, the disease perspective, considers how alterations in biological functioning cause some of the person's difficulties. The disease perspective considers *what the person has*. Persons who have borderline personality disorder frequently suffer from treatable illnesses, like major depressive disorder or bipolar disorder, which bring about severe mood changes, depression, irritability, and other intensely uncomfortable mood states that not only are extremely impairing in themselves, but make it impossible for these individuals to benefit from psychological treatments for these other problems. We reviewed some of the research that suggests that persons with the borderline diagnosis have subtle alterations in brain functioning that are responsible for some of their problems, such as their difficulties modulating mood. These problems, caused by biological factors, require medical treatments aimed at correcting or compensating for the alterations in functioning: medications.

We also reviewed how extremes of temperament contribute to the problems of persons who have BPD. The dimensional perspective considers how an individual's personality characteristics, which vary from person to person, determine *who the person is*; persons with this diagnosis are on the extreme end of the tendency to react to difficulties by experiencing unpleasant emotions like anxiety, depression, and anger. Whereas some people have a more placid, unflappable personality and can take problems in stride, these individuals react quickly and negatively to stresses and setbacks. We also discussed how individuals with this diagnosis are unsettled and fragile in their sense of self, seeing themselves as damaged or defective, which leads them to cling to others in unhealthy ways that usually have the effect of destroying the support they need and the intimacy they crave. The art and science of psychodynamic psychotherapy focuses on helping patients see themselves more objectively and to analyze where their emotions come from and why they react as they do to people and situations.

Persons who have borderline personality disorder invariably develop maladaptive and self-destructive behaviors to deal with their extreme emotional pain. They learn how alcohol or drugs can numb their pain, and how self-mutilation can refocus their distress to bearable physical rather than unbearable psychic pain. These behaviors, *what the person does,* become entrenched and entrapping, persisting and returning to plague the person whenever she encounters problems. Treatments that extinguish these maladaptive behaviors and replace them with healthier coping patterns help with this set of problems, such as dialectical behavioral therapy and specific treatments for problems like addictions and eating disorders.

Last, we reviewed how many of the problems these individuals have can be understood by listening to their life story, that *what the person has encountered* makes a significant contribution to his problems. As children, persons who have BPD lived in what Linehan has called an "invalidating" environment, where their feelings were discounted or ignored, causing them to develop a damaged view of themselves as defective or even evil. Much too often, this is because of childhood abuse, frequently sexual abuse, but sometimes it results from more subtle forces, such as a mismatch between the person's extremes of temperament and a less-than-accommodating parenting style at home. Again, psychotherapy helps the patient correct this distorted perception of himself, heal his damaged identity, make peace with the past, and put it behind him.

A successful treatment plan addresses these problems one by one and will necessarily be multifaceted and require a team of several professionals who bring different skill sets to the effort.

Many, perhaps most, people who have borderline personality disorder will need ongoing psychiatric treatment (that is, treatment from a physician), or at the least a psychiatric evaluation. The purpose of this intervention will be to identify psychiatric illnesses that can be alleviated by treatment with medications. The symptoms of these illnesses will interfere with treatment for the other problems these persons have and will usually need to be among the first of the interventions put in place for them.

Also at the top of the treatment agenda will be intervention to interrupt self-destructive behaviors. Behaviors like self-mutilation and repeated suicide attempts generate continual crises for the person who has BPD, for her loved ones, and for the treatment team. Constant interruptions to ongoing psychotherapeutic treatment to manage these crises will prevent the patient from addressing subtler, slower-to-change problems like temperamental extremes and difficulties in emotional modulation. Also, until the individual has developed better behavioral control and healthier, more adaptive coping mechanisms, she will be unable to address painful past events without needing to fall back on these maladaptive behavioral patterns; making peace with the past grinds to a halt. Cognitive behavioral therapy and especially dialectical behavioral therapy have been developed especially for the purpose of interrupting these behaviors.

There is also evidence that other forms of psychotherapy specifically developed for these patients (transference-based psychotherapy for borderline personality disorder and mentalization- and schema-based therapies) can be effective for this purpose; clearly psychotherapy that doesn't directly address and plan for the management of these behaviors, like traditional psychodynamic psychotherapy, is not usually effective. The person may also need treatment for other kinds of self-destructive behaviors like addiction or an eating disorder. Any and all of these behavioral problems must be under good control before the individual can move on to the self-appraisal needed to achieve an enhanced understanding of herself and her past.

Only when the symptoms of psychiatric illness are under control and self-destructive behaviors have been extinguished will the person be able to move on to more fundamental change. This will also require specialized psychotherapy, as we have discussed.

Obviously, then, the path to treatment success for borderline personality disorder is a rather long and winding one, requiring perseverance above all. We know, however, that treatment pays off. As we've emphasized throughout this book, borderline personality disorder, once thought to be practically untreatable, is now considered a good prognosis psychiatric disorder.

CHAPTER 13

Themes and Variations

In this chapter, we explore some of the differences that exist between various groups of people in how borderline personality disorder affects individuals. First, we look at the different ways in which men and women express the symptoms and behaviors of the disorder. Though most experts have concluded that the similarities outweigh the differences, the variances are significant enough to bear discussion.

Although the term *personality disorder* is usually applied exclusively to adults and not to children and adolescents, in whom personality is still developing, various difficulties that appear to be precursors to the diagnosis can be seen in younger people, for whom standard treatment approaches are less effective, necessitating modifications of the techniques.

Finally, another set of differences that bears discussing is the way the disorder varies among different cultural groups.

Gender Differences

Borderline personality is usually reported to be a disorder that affects predominantly women. Although many researchers have indeed found this to be the case, some have not. Most studies that have found this preponderance have been done in clinical settings (psychiatric clinics or hospitals), wherein about three-quarters of patients with this diagnosis are women. The problem with these data is the known fact that women tend to seek out mental health treatment more readily than men. Therefore, since more women seek treatment than men, proportionately more women will often be seen in studies done in clinical settings, and the study results may not reflect the true proportion of individuals in the community who have the disorder. One way around this problem is to interview random individuals in the general population rather than persons who have sought treatment; several studies have attempted to do this. But this approach has its problems too, the main one being that many persons need to be interviewed in the general population (usually many thousands) to get accurate numbers on relatively uncommon illnesses. Also, researchers inevitably have to rely on interviewers with less professional training and use simplified and relatively unsophisticated questionnaires. One research project that took this approach found borderline personality disorder to be equally common in men and women.[1] Another study took the approach of asking parents about their children being treated for borderline personality disorder, specifically parents who visited the Web site of the National Education Alliance for Borderline Personality Disorder. These researchers found that although men with the diagnosis were just as likely to have been hospitalized or to have spent time living in a psychiatric halfway house, they were much less likely than women with the diagnosis to have been in DBT or treated with medication.[2] They tended to have had more treatment for drug abuse problems. The researchers concluded that there must be some barrier to men getting into treatment; perhaps the diagnosis is under-recognized in men, and therefore appropriate treatment is not offered.

Several studies have investigated whether there are differences in the patterns of symptoms seen in men versus women with the borderline diagnosis. The findings are fairly consistent over these studies, which consistently indicate that more men than women who have borderline personality disorder have problems with addiction and are more likely to have a significant history of antisocial behaviors (pervasive problems with lying, irresponsibility and dishonesty, criminal activities, physical aggressiveness toward others, and lack of remorse). On the other hand, more women than men have eating disorders, and they are more likely to have been the victims of sexual abuse or assault and to have developed symptoms of PTSD.[3,4,5] It has been argued, however, that these patterns are seen in the general population as well; that is, addiction and antisocial problems are more common in men, and eating disorders and sexual victimization are more common in women generally, not only in those who have been diagnosed with borderline personality disorder.

It has been proposed that these differences simply reflect the particulars ways in which men and women deal with emotional pain. Women have been described as more vulnerable to what have been called *internalizing disorders*, tending to direct their emotional distress inward, while men more commonly develop *externalizing disorders*, where they project distress outward into the environment.

As far as the features of borderline personality disorder (chronic emotional pain, problems with emotional modulation and impulsivity, and all the others we've reviewed), differences in symptom patterns between men and women have not clearly emerged in the research literature.

The bottom line, then, is that men and women who have borderline personality disorder are more alike than different as far as the borderline features, but they have different rates of complicating problems that reflect the pattern seen in men versus women generally. The most significant finding, perhaps, is that the complicating disorders seen in men (their problems with alcoholism, drug abuse, and antisocial behaviors) are what tend to bring them into contact with the systems of care where their borderline features tend to get missed (addiction facilities and the criminal justice system), and they are less likely to get specialized treatment for the personality disorder that underlies their other problems.

Borderline Personality Disorder in Adolescence

Does it make sense to speak of a "personality disorder" in adolescents? After all, adolescence is generally thought of as the time in a person's life when his personality is undergoing a great deal of change and development. The DSM cautions:

Personality Disorder categories may be applied to children or adolescents in those relatively unusual instances in which the individual's particular maladaptive personality traits appear to be pervasive, persistent, and unlikely to be limited to a particular developmental stage or an episode of an Axis I disorder. It should be recognized that the traits of a Personality Disorder that appear in childhood will often not persist unchanged into adult life.[6]

Although diagnoses are meant to indicate a focus of treatment and clinical attention rather than label anyone, many mental health professionals remain extremely reluctant to make personality disorder diagnoses in adolescents, even more so in children, often for fear of just that: assigning a stigmatizing label that may turn out to be incorrect. Despite this understandable reluctance, we know that many psychiatric problems become apparent and can be readily diagnosed in adolescence; mood disorders are a good example. Also, as you realize by now, borderline personality disorder is much more than a personality problem. So, almost as a compromise, it is common to refer to children and adolescents as having borderline "traits," but to reserve the diagnosis of "personality disorder" for individuals over 18 years old, except in extremely clear-cut cases.

Although, as the DSM indicates, borderline traits will not necessarily persist into adulthood, adolescents with these characteristics are more likely to be subsequently diagnosed with a personality disorder as well as another comorbid disorder, such as a mood disorder. Therefore, these traits should certainly not be ignored in the hopes that they will simply go away, because they are often an indicator of psychiatric problems of some kind. Rather, the clinician is presented with an opportunity to make a real impact on the young person's future mental health; there is evidence that identifying and treating these problems at an earlier age rather than waiting until the person is an adult can reduce the future incidence of both personality disorders and their common comorbidities (such as eating disorders and addictions).

But how to identify borderline personality characteristics in children and adolescents? Many adolescents go through a rebellious stage as part of their normal development, in which their sense of identity and emotions fluctuate greatly. Their relationships are unstable and constantly reconfiguring. They suffer from a significant burden of the hubris of youth, frequently feeling indestructible and thus making impulsive and poor decisions. How does one differentiate a normal developmental stage from the germs of psychiatric disorder? There are three indicators: the severity of these problems, their persistence, and the distress they cause.

By severity, we mean situations where symptoms would be unusual even in the sometimes tumultuous emotional life of an adolescent. Suicidal behaviors, self-mutilation, chronic feelings of emptiness (as opposed to the romanticized ennui) are all red flags that something more serious is occurring that the normal developmental process doesn't adequately explain. All too often, parents are tempted to see these symptoms too as a "phase." We are suggesting not that every adolescent who states he feels empty must urgently have a psychiatric evaluation, only that these symptoms may be an indicator of something more troublesome and therefore deserve special attention and close monitoring. In addition, extreme degrees of any symptoms that characterize borderline personality disorder (that is, impulsivity that actually threatens a person's life, or anger episodes that put others at risk) certainly warrant further attention. Most adolescents resent the implication that there is anything "wrong" with them or that they are "different." But seeking help when these danger signs are present in an adolescent is not harmful or "getting in their business"; rather, it is a call to preventive arms and, quite frankly, well within the purview of the parents' responsibility to look out for their child.

Another indicator of serious problems may be the persistence of less worrisome and more subtle symptoms for more than a few months. As adolescents dip into the often turbulent waters of the teenage social scene, they may be extremely popular one month and then, for no discernible reason, find themselves at the bottom of the social heap. This may lead to perceptions of emptiness and loneliness and seeming emotional instability. But despite the adolescent's common perception that this will last forever, these symptoms do resolve, and moods do stabilize. If this does not occur, however, it may indicate something amiss in the developmental trajectory that requires addressing.

The final, and possibly most important, factor to watch for is the level of dysfunction caused by these symptoms. Fortunately, this is usually easy to spot—if an adolescent has alienated himself from friends and family due to severe mood problems, if grades suddenly start to drop precipitously or if he frequently feels so empty that he avoids school or friends, then help of some sort is clearly warranted.

Unfortunately, more often than not, the people trying to help fix the problem (parents, teachers, friends) are perceived by the adolescent to *be* the problem. The tendency to see one's problems as the result of uncaring or overtly hostile others is typical of individuals who have borderline personality disorder. Nevertheless, assessment and, if needed, treatment by a qualified mental health professional can not only help put the adolescent back on track, but can help the entire family breathe a sigh of relief.

In terms of the symptoms and behaviors, adolescents who have BPD actually don't differ significantly from their adult counterparts—except that the symptoms and behaviors can be much more dramatic and intense. Although adults have sometimes suffered the consequences of their actions and developed some coping skills to deal with the outside world (however maladaptive), adolescents live in a somewhat protected world. All teenagers are in ideological flux, let alone those with borderline personality disorder. As such, they tend to be more impulsive, more distressed, and more afraid of loss than their adult counterparts. They quickly flip from one emotional extreme to the other. Clinicians are frequently called to treat an adolescent with "severe bipolar affective disorder" who turns out to in fact have borderline personality disorder.

Despite their symptoms resembling those of their adult counterparts, adolescents who have borderline personality disorder frequently require somewhat different treatment approaches and have different issues that need to be addressed.

As with all children and adolescents, these persons are typically far more embedded in the family's home life. Family involvement is always a crucial component in treatment because the family is usually the adolescent's single most important support system (or stressor, and frequently both).

Similarly, some therapists neglect to focus adequately on the patient's social world, preferring one-to-one therapy. Adults who have borderline personality disorder may go to work and be able to live individual lives outside their work. They have significant others but typically also pursue their own interests. Even those people who have BPD have some sense of mastery over their surroundings and some individual identity, flawed though it may be. Adolescents, on the other hand, typically define themselves *only* in relation to their social surroundings—even if they strive to be an individual or different from everyone else, it is their "differentness" that defines them. For nearly everyone in high school—the social outcast or the quarterback—the social role essentially defines every aspect of their experience: who they hang out with, what they do in and after school, who they could date, and so on. Ignoring the social pressures and environments in which adolescents are so fundamentally enmeshed makes treatment much more difficult, if not impossible.

For these and many other reasons, adult treatment approaches have been modified specifically for children and adolescents with traits of borderline personality disorder; some entirely new approaches have even been developed.

A specialized form of dialectical behavioral therapy (DBT) has been created for adolescents that we would like to discuss in some detail.[7] Many of the underlying tenets and the framework of DBT with adolescents are the same as with adults, but there are also significant differences. With adults, for example, the therapist spends a large amount of time describing the dialectic of borderline personality disorder and having the patient own the illness as a first step. Along the way, patients must constantly reaffirm their desire to improve through contracting to abstain from certain behaviors. They establish contracts promising to use certain skills to avoid problematic situations, based on their understanding that they behave in a way consistent with borderline personality disorder.

In adolescents, this approach often doesn't work because the adolescent typically has not experienced enough adverse consequences of their actions to understand that they are at the root of their own problems. Instead they have often externalized the source of difficulty—they would be fine if only it wasn't for her meddling and difficult family, her horrible teacher, her aloof boyfriend, and so on. Many adolescents see therapy itself as a source of difficulty rather than help and consequently are typically more or less coerced into therapy by their parents. Requiring the adolescent to take ownership of her illness and make a commitment to improve may abort therapy before it has even started. In these situations, the therapist typically must take a step back and deal with individual behaviors and problems rather than requiring acceptance of the illness as a whole. Problems must sometimes be reframed—if the therapy is a problem, then successfully completing it will alleviate that problem. If the person's aloof boyfriend is the cause of her constant consternation (rather than her clinginess and emotional dependence on him), then setting up more strict boundaries and structure in their relationship will help him be more regularly attentive. If a particular teacher "hates" her and is the cause of her failing school, then reducing the attention drawn to herself by problem behaviors as well as "proving him wrong" by getting better grades are alternative ways of making her point rather than screaming in the classroom.

The family is much more involved in DBT with adolescents than with adults. Parents are often required to attend skills training meetings, just as the patient is. In these training sessions, they all learn the same skills for emotional regulation, distress tolerance, interpersonal effectiveness, and mindfulness. They are also taught specific responses (sometimes in the form of an actual written script) to common stressful events at home. These responses are highly personalized to the family's specific experiences with their problematic family member. The groups serve multiple purposes. The first is education about the disorder. The family is taught that borderline personality disorder, just like bipolar disorder or diabetes, is not under the patient's control. Though the person who has BPD is being taught to modulate her feelings and control her behavior through therapy, it is not her "fault" that she behaves the way she does. Parents must also be educated to realize that the adolescent's painful emotions are at the bottom of her behaviors, not maliciousness. Adolescents who have borderline traits feel frighteningly out of control and in a great deal of distress when they are acting out. Their manipulative tendencies are not something they do to "get" their parents, but are a sign of just how much distress they are in. Also, family members must learn how to modulate their own emotional responses to the teenager. The behaviors of persons who have borderline personality disorder trigger intense anger, frustration, and other negative feelings in those around them. Acting on these feelings typically leads family members to respond to the individual in ways that exacerbate and prolong, rather than alleviate, the stressful situation at hand. Learning coping techniques to minimize these negative responses can be extremely helpful in terminating negative situations before they get out of control. In addition, the genetic and biological underpinnings of borderline personality disorder are relevant. Other members of the family may also have borderline personality symptoms and traits, though often to a less severe degree. Family members often find that mastering the skills they learn in these sessions is extremely helpful in modulating their own negative behaviors and improving their other interpersonal relationships.

The skills taught in adolescent DBT are somewhat different than those in traditional DBT as well. In addition to emotional regulation, distress tolerance, interpersonal effectiveness, and mindfulness (mindfulness is particularly important for this population), the adolescent and his family must also master skills of "walking the middle path." This module was specifically created to address the relationship between adolescents and their families, typically their parents. Some of the most destabilizing factors in the relationship among members of these families are power struggles. Although the parents typically feel themselves to be in control in the family, the adolescent can wrest it away from them in many situations. This can come in many forms—rebellion, anger, yelling, crying, manipulation, and even suicidal behaviors. In fact, many persons who have BPD will, in retrospect, admit that suicidal attempts were carried out with the intended goal of gaining some control within the family.

The point of walking the middle path is similar to Linehan's concept of the emotional dialectic, recognizing and accepting opposites when it comes to feelings but striving for a healthy synthesis of these contradictory positions. However, the approach is expanded beyond managing one's own emotional conflicts and applied to solving conflicts in everyday life between family members. A person is encouraged to constantly "strive for the middle," avoiding the extremes of emotions and behaviors that pollute relationships. Teens are counseled to avoid thinking of their parents as all good or all bad, all punishing or all rewarding. Similarly, parents are advised to find a balance between punishment and reward—to be neither too harsh nor too permissive with their child. During interactions between family members, each is counseled to constantly ask themselves, "What is the middle path here? What is the contrary position to how I see the other person right now?" Parents are encouraged to find a middle path between being too permissive versus too strict with their teen, making light of problematic behaviors versus making too much of typical adolescent behavior, and being overprotective versus forcing independence too soon.

Walking the middle path also focuses on validation. Through therapy, individuals learn to balance validating themselves and their behavior with striving to change. The phrase "you're doing the best that you can (with the skills you have), but now you must do better" is frequently quoted by therapists. The person learns that self-blame is only useful if it inspires change—if, instead, it leads to feeling worse about oneself and therefore to an increase in negative behaviors, it is destructive. With that view in mind, individuals who have BPD are taught to go over past experiences, not in a judging or blaming way, but with the view that they did the absolute best job they could in that situation—but that now, their task is to look for things that they can work on and possibly change for future situations. This viewpoint ameliorates the person's negative feelings about herself by tempering confrontation with acceptance. The adolescent can review her experiences and feelings (rather than avoiding them because she is too full of self-loathing and pain) with the goal of looking for opportunities to improve.

Parents often have a difficult time accepting this message. Validating a destructive behavior as "the best you could have done at the time" is such a foreign concept to many that this approach can initially be met with much resistance. Often, such a reservoir of frustration and anger has built up within the parents because of their child's problem behaviors that any validation is just unacceptable. It may seem that the therapist is actually encouraging the behavior, or demanding that the parents give up control. Parents must learn that validating an adolescent's feelings and point of view is not the same as agreeing with them; rather, it recognizes some internal point that has some merit (even if that merit is based on sometimes emotional and irrational principles). Parents learn that validating behavior and feelings is critical to maintaining a healthy relationship with the adolescent—the alternative is either to harshly punish or to withdraw, both of which are particularly terrifying to the person who has BPD and therefore lead to increased negative behavior. According to this program, validation of the adolescent's feelings by parents shows that

- they are listening
- they understand
- they are being nonjudgmental
- they care about the relationship
- conflict and disagreement is possible without disruptive emotional intensity

Although it often feels foreign initially, validating feelings and behaviors (tempered, remember, with the recognition of the need to figure out how to do better next time) can be incredibly healing to the relationship.

This process of validation is a two-way street, and the adolescent is helped to accept and understand her parents' feelings and behaviors; in fact, she must learn to accept them, even if she does not fully understand. Parents may have done things or expressed feelings that seem silly or malicious to the adolescent, and young people often have a great deal of difficulty forgiving the perceived sins of their parents. Learning to see things from the parents' perspective is often a first step to being able to validate *them* as individuals. The point is to recognize that both members of a disagreement are human beings, with their own perspectives and feelings. Just because you disagree does not mean that your viewpoint is the only correct one; nor does it mean that the other person is delusional and not making any sense. Being able to comprehend, or at least tolerate, each other's behavior and subsequently validate their point of view can eliminate power struggles and encourage compromise, the essence of walking the middle path.

International and Cross-Cultural Considerations

Studies to determine if there are differences in the prevalence or symptoms of persons who have borderline personality disorder in different countries and among different ethnic populations are in their infancy. There is clearly a big problem with making accurate diagnoses when the researchers and the patients are not from the same ethnic or cultural group. It should come as no surprise, then, that surveying international and cross-cultural differences among those diagnosed with borderline personality disorder often yields confusing, and sometimes even contradictory, data.

One expert proposes that "indirect evidence, deriving from cross-cultural differences in the prevalence of symptoms such as [suicidal gestures], suicide, antisocial behavior, and substance abuse, strongly suggests that [the disorder] is more frequent in modern than in traditional societies."[8] But there is still little direct evidence to support this contention. He hypothesizes, based on an understanding of the work of Marsha Linehan, that "children who later develop BPD have a constitutionally determined emotional instability that requires more buffering from parents, who are needed to help modulate and control the child's dysphoric emotions. The modern world, which demands greater individual autonomy, and which allows less dependence on or attachment to others, interferes with the ability of children who have stronger emotional needs to obtain sufficient care from their families. Borderline personality disorder is most likely to develop when these temperamental, parental, and social risk factors are present at the same time."

A survey of 1,583 patients discharged from a Bronx hospital with a psychiatric diagnosis showed that, among white and black patients, at least three times more women than men were diagnosed with borderline personality disorder—but this difference was not observed among the Hispanics in the sample, where the gender distribution was about even.[9] A subsequent study looked at 606 psychiatric patients (a mixture of previously admitted inpatients and treated outpatients) diagnosed with a personality disorder. This study found that the proportion of personality disorder patients who had BPD was significantly higher in the Hispanic subjects.[10]

These authors proposed several possible reasons for this difference. One reason, they stated, may be that many Hispanics need to adjust to a new cultural norm when they come to the United States, leading to an identity diffusion that could have destabilized a previously mild personality disorder. This same explanation (inherent cultural differences) can also, however, lead to an alternative conclusion: that Anglo psychiatrists, unfamiliar with the norms of Latin culture, may perceive some behaviors as pathological and representing a personality disorder, when they are perfectly acceptable within the framework of the person's culture. When further analysis was carried out in an attempt to see if the pattern of borderline symptoms differed among the ethnic groups, Hispanics diagnosed with borderline personality disorder had a greater prevalence of the symptoms of intense anger, mood instability, and unstable relationships. The authors noted, however, that "within Puerto Rican culture, men are permitted to be more emotional than women and to exhibit strong emotions such as anger, aggressiveness, and sexual attraction," characteristics that are seen as pathological in Anglo-American men.

They also make note of a cultural phenomenon within some Hispanic communities called *ataque de nervios*. Ataques can be triggered by a stressful event relating to the family, including death of a loved one, conflicts with a spouse or children, or witnessing an accident involving a family member. Manifestations of ataques de nervios can include "uncontrollable shouting, attacks of crying, trembling, heat in the chest rising into the head, and verbal or physical aggression,"[11] emotional reactions that, although they are a common expression of distress within this culture, are likely to be judged as overly dramatic and diagnostic of a personality disorder by clinicians unfamiliar with the culture.

FOR AN EXTENDED PERIOD, psychiatrists in Great Britain were resistant to the concept of borderline personality disorder as a valid diagnostic entity, and consequently, the diagnosis was rarely made in British patients even as late as the 1980s. With the advent of the American DSM-III in the early 1980s and also the development of the Diagnostic Interview for Borderlines (DIB), an interview tool designed by a prominent American expert in borderline personality disorder, Dr. John Gunderson of the McLean Hospital, especially for the purpose of making the diagnosis, investigators in Britain set out to answer the question that eventually became the title of the journal article that reported their findings, "Are There Borderlines in Britain?"[12] One clinician examined forty-seven psychiatric inpatients using the DIB and found a 14.9 percent incidence of borderline personality disorder. When a different clinician used the DSM criteria, only 8.5 percent of the patients were diagnosed with borderline personality disorder (all of whom also met criteria on the DIB). What diagnoses had the British psychiatrists taking care of these patients made? All patients had received a personality disorder diagnosis, including some categories not used in the United States, like "explosive," "neurotic," "immature," and "inadequate."

The conclusions reached by these authors were ambivalent to say the least. On the one hand, they admitted that (1) persons who fit the borderline personality disorder description (as evaluated by three American mental health workers using the DSM-III and DIB) do exist in England; and that (2) these persons received ICD (*International Statistical Classification of Diseases*) personality disorder diagnoses from the British psychiatrists. But on the other hand, they continued to question whether "borderline personality" was a real category:

> It remains an open question as to whether borderline and other per-
> sonality disorders can be reliably differentiated from each other and
> have valid and separate concepts . . . One tentatively might conclude
> from this that a patient identified by a British psychiatrist as having hys-
> terical or explosive personality disorder, especially with an additional
> depressive component, would very likely be identified as having border-
> line personality disorder by an American psychiatrist . . . Many border-
> line patients are best viewed and treated as variants of mood-disordered
> patients who respond to their (subjectively unpleasant) dysphoria with
> hysterical and self-destructive behaviors.

This had been the thinking of many American psychiatrists until shortly before this time, and this controversy illustrates why so little research on the disorder was done outside a few academic centers in both the United States and Britain for the next several decades, leading to a long delay in the development of effective treatments.

Britain has, however, clearly caught up now. For a time, there were even National Health Service hospitals established specifically for the treatment of patients who had severe personality disorders, including borderline personality disorder.

IN JAPAN, the diagnosis of borderline personality disorder was not in general use among psychiatrists in the 1980s either. In fact there was something of a diagnostic tradition in Japan of "one patient, one diagnosis," so that personality disorder diagnoses of any type were uncommonly made in Japanese patients. A group of Japanese clinicians used basically the same methods as their British colleagues and administered the DIB and applied DSM criteria to eighty-five women between the ages of 18 and 30 who were receiving outpatient treatment. Thirty-eight percent of these women met criteria for the diagnosis of borderline personality disorder. In addition, they had the same common cooccurring illnesses as their Western counterparts (mood disorders, eating disorders, and substance use disorders). The pattern of symptoms of these individuals was only slightly different from that found in studies of American persons who had BPD. For example, fewer patients had drug abuse problems, but there is a much lower prevalence of drug abuse in the Japanese population as a whole. Also, "intense unstable relationships" were more common, but being "socially isolated, loner" was less common. The authors explain that women in this age group are far more likely to live at home with their parents than were their American counterparts, leading to more intense power struggles and problematic relationships.[13] The authors concluded, "there are indeed borderline personality disorder patients in Japan [and] . . . their clinical picture is no different from that of American patients."

THE CHINESE have their own version of the ICD and DSM called the *Chinese Classification of Mental Disorders* (CCMD), currently in its third iteration. Despite it being intended to be similar to the DSM and ICD, the committee responsible for developing it rejected the concept of borderline personality disorder, instead adopting the diagnosis of "impulsive personality disorder" (IPD). According to one Chinese author, "It was argued that the [borderline] diagnosis is a vague construct that lacks precise boundaries, and some of its diagnostic features (e.g., fear of abandonment, chronic feelings of emptiness) are not appropriate culturally when used in China."[14] In contrast with the borderline diagnosis, the diagnosis of IPD requires the trait of impulsivity (whereas this is one of many criteria in the DSM) but omits several DSM criteria such as chronic feelings of emptiness, fear of abandonment, or transient psychotic phenomena. No validation of the diagnostic construct of impulsive personality disorder has been carried out, and therefore its criteria are based on clinical experience rather than evidence.

Despite this refusal to include the diagnosis in the CCMD, many studies similar to the ones discussed above used DSM criteria to examine Chinese patients. Although none of these studies published their results in a paper called "Are There Borderlines in China?" the answer to that question is clearly "Yes." Also despite the official denial of the usefulness of the diagnostic category in the Chinese, there have been, as of this writing, more research articles on borderline personality disorder published by Chinese authors about Chinese patients than on any other personality disorder, with sixteen original studies, fifteen review articles and eight case reports published between 1979 and 2008.[15] It appears that, although not officially recognized, more and more researchers are acknowledging the presence of BPD in the Chinese population, and that the prevalence (at least according to one study) is roughly the same as in the United States.

DUE TO THE DIAGNOSTIC VARIABILITY and disagreement on the criteria for diagnosing personality disorders worldwide, the World Health Organization is attempting to develop standardized diagnostic criteria for these conditions that can be applied equally to different cultures and that are less likely to yield inaccurate results because a researcher is biased by a lack of familiarity with the patient's culture. The WHO has developed the International Personality Disorders Examination, an interview administered by psychiatrists that corresponds to ICD and DSM criteria for personality disorders, and work is beginning that will determine whether it will accomplish this lofty goal.

Due to the structured nature of the interview (examiners are taught to lead with certain questions to collect symptoms for various disorders, though they can trail off in other directions as appropriate), it was thought that the results would be much more uniform than subjective diagnoses. In the first study of this instrument, 716 patients throughout the world (from India, Switzerland, the Netherlands, Britain, Germany, Kenya, the United States, Norway, Japan, and Australia) were examined. The overall percentage of people diagnosed with borderline personality disorder was 14.9 percent, and the inter-rater reliability, a measure of how frequently different clinicians who interviewed the same patients made the same diagnosis, was 0.8 (in statistical terms, this is considered "outstanding" reliability). Though this paper did not do any analyses to determine percentages for individual countries, the overall percentage corresponds roughly with what is seen in the United States.

Increasing numbers of research studies indicate that some people in every culture and country have borderline personality disorder, and that they do not differ significantly from one another as far as their symptoms, behaviors, and co-occurring disorders. However, the ways in which those cultures address those traits may be different. Chinese psychiatry continues to insist that borderline personality disorder does not exist in China. It appears, then, that the key difference in borderline personality across different cultures is how accurately it is diagnosed and therefore how it is treated.

IV

How to Cope,
How to Help

CHAPTER 14

If You've Been Diagnosed with Borderline Personality Disorder

One of the necessary steps in the process of getting this book published was having an expert on borderline personality disorder review the first draft. The reviewer (whose identity is unknown to the authors) is given a series of questions that essentially ask him or her to weigh in on the scientific accuracy of what's been written and give a "thumbs up" or "thumbs down" on whether the book should be published. The last question is always something along the lines of, "How might the manuscript be improved?" Our reviewer responded:

> I would like to see a sense of optimism and hope be present in the final draft. More recently, the disorder has been called "the good prognosis diagnosis" and it is important to include that in writings in this decade.

We'll repeat that for emphasis: *the disorder has been called "the good prognosis diagnosis."* We can state that quite confidently thanks to about a decade of research on treatment that unequivocally shows this to be true. Nearly 90 percent of persons with the borderline personality disorder diagnosis who entered the decade-long McLean Hospital study that we have cited repeatedly throughout this book attained a sustained remission from their symptoms, defined as at least four years of no longer meeting DSM diagnostic criteria for the diagnosis. A substantial proportion of these patients recovered completely, defined as "having an emotionally sustaining relationship with a close friend or life partner or spouse, and being able to work or go to school consistently, competently, and on a full-time basis."[1] All these subjects had entered the study while on an inpatient unit, meaning that they were starting during a time of severe symptoms, "from the bottom." When you consider that a substantial number of persons with this diagnosis are never hospitalized, it's probably safe to say that this study *underestimates* the proportion of all patients with this diagnosis who achieve a sustained recovery.

Diagnosis, Diagnosis, Diagnosis

You've likely heard that old chestnut about the three most important factors in determining the value of a piece of real estate: "location, location, location." There is a similar truism about the most important factors in determining the correctness of a treatment plan—we've titled this section after them. More specifically, getting the *correct* diagnosis is key.

If there's one thing that we hope you've learned about borderline personality disorder from this book so far, it's that this diagnosis encompasses a complex combination of symptoms and behavioral problems that intertwine and interact with each other in myriad ways. It is never an easy problem to diagnose. Because of these complexities and how challenging it is to devise an effective treatment plan for this disorder, even many professionals have misconceptions about it or simply haven't the training or experience needed to plan appropriate treatment. Some diagnose *any* patient who has "cutting" behaviors with borderline personality disorder. But self-mutilation is a behavior, not a diagnosis, and it can occur in many different types of psychiatric problems. Skilled psychotherapists recognize that some individuals who have never developed cutting behaviors, who go to work every day and function quite normally in many different ways, nevertheless have this diagnosis and benefit greatly from dialectical behavioral therapy (DBT). We have seen patients referred to us for the treatment of a mood disorder whose problems with emotional dysregulation were actually due to borderline personality disorder. And we've seen patients who have been given the borderline personality diagnosis whose "personality disorder" is "cured" by treating them with medications effective for bipolar disorder. So how do you go about making sure *your* diagnosis is correct?

The way that medical professionals deal with complicated problems is to get advice from other professionals with different areas of expertise. For the patient, this means being willing to pursue recommendations for consultations. If your psychiatrist recommends that you start seeing a psychotherapist, or your psychotherapist recommends a psychiatric consultation, then take this advice and do so.

The best way to get a useful consultation is to come to the appointment with a well-articulated question for the consultant. "My therapist and I want to know if I might have a mood disorder"; "My psychiatrist and I are wondering if psychotherapy might be a helpful addition to my treatment for bipolar disorder." Your therapist may want to get a consultation from another psychotherapist with more experience in treating persons who have borderline personality disorder, in which case the consultation question might be, "Would DBT be beneficial for me?" On the other hand, the perfect way to render a consultation next to useless for everyone is to simply show up at the consultation appointment and say, "My doctor said I had to see you, but I don't think I need to." Another counterproductive approach is to come to the consultation with the question already answered, such as with a statement like "I'm here because I need medication."

A consultation will be more helpful if the consultant has information about you from the referring professional; a referral letter outlining your treatment history will be an invaluable time saver.

Consulting with a psychotherapist will usually require more than just a single appointment, especially if there is a question of a personality disorder. Several appointments will be necessary before a therapist will get to know you well enough to begin formulating the best way to think about a psychological approach to your symptoms.

Remember that there is a difference between appropriate consultation and "doctor shopping," that is, seeing one professional after another until you find one who tells you what you want to hear. Psychiatric diagnosis is a process of narrowing down diagnostic possibilities and refining the diagnostic formulation; making too many fresh starts interrupts this process and just keeps everybody guessing. Teamwork is key.

Assembling Your Treatment Team

As you've undoubtedly learned from reading this book so far, many aspects of the treatment of borderline personality disorder are quite specialized. Minimum requirements for your treatment would be a psychiatrist skilled in treating mood disorders and a therapist experienced in treating patients with borderline personality disorder.

DBT is currently the most thoroughly studied and widely available treatment approach for treating the most problematic and dangerous symptoms of borderline personality disorder, self-destructive behaviors like cutting and suicidal behaviors. Without getting these problems under control, real improvement remains out of reach. Ideally, therefore, your therapist should be part of a practice that offers DBT, which will consist of individual therapy and group sessions (reread chapter 11 if you need to refresh your knowledge of the different components of DBT).

In our experience, it takes a rather special person to work with persons who have this diagnosis, a therapist with perhaps a bit more patience and unflappability than most. Since DBT is a treatment approach used almost exclusively for persons who have BPD, seeking out a practice that offers DBT is usually an excellent way to find a therapeutic team with the specialized training, experience, and professional interest in treating borderline personality disorder. Fortunately, the number of mental health practices and centers that offer DBT is constantly growing, and many larger metropolitan areas have several practices.

Some extraordinary psychiatrists may be *both* excellent mood disorder psychopharmacologists and trained and experienced in DBT, but they are surely few and far between, because these are two different skill sets, both of which require long training periods and staying up-to-date with an enormous amount of varied research. Most psychiatrists these days are either primarily psychopharmacologists or primarily psychotherapists for this reason. However, most mental health practices that offer DBT will have a psychiatrist or psychiatrists who work closely with the psychotherapists and thus will have professionals with all the skills required to effectively treat this disorder.

Therapists trained in DBT will often strictly limit the number of patients they take into their caseload whom they treat with DBT. Persons requiring DBT may thus make up only a small proportion of their patients. This is because the treatment of persons who have this diagnosis is often quite demanding and time intensive. In appendix A, we list several national resources that will be helpful in locating DBT specialists near you.

You may have a relationship with a therapist who does not have training in DBT and wonder if you should switch therapists to get into a DBT program. This is a difficult question to answer. On the one hand, effective psychological treatment requires a long-term relationship with a trusted therapist, and if you already have this valuable asset, you may want to hold onto it. But on the other hand, if you decide that despite your and your therapist's best efforts in treatment, progress in stopping self-destructive behaviors has been an elusive goal, it makes sense to explore other options. Sometimes an effective compromise in this situation will be staying with your therapist for individual therapy and supplementing that treatment with a DBT skills-building group. Your therapist should be willing to discuss these options with you; the discussion may be more productive if you've done some homework, such as finding the names of therapists or practices that provide DBT. A consultation with another professional with more specialized knowledge may be the only way to sort through these issues.

HEALTH CARE FINANCING in the United States is evolving rapidly as this is being written, and fortunately, easier and more affordable access to mental health services appears to be part of this evolution. That said, we have a long way to go, and specialized mental health care can still be difficult to obtain. Most medical insurance plans provide mental health treatment as "carved out" treatment, meaning that there are often separate phone numbers to call and personnel who administer mental health benefits. Frequently, these personnel are not even employees of the company on your medical insurance card but work for a separate company called a *managed care organization*. All of this means that finding out what is covered by your insurance can be a bureaucratic nightmare. It is often easier to find the treating professionals first, then ask them whether they accept your insurance.

If you don't have health insurance (and hopefully, the evolution we referred to above means that the number who don't will be steadily decreasing over time), there are often hospital-affiliated practices or subsidized community mental health centers that will provide treatment on a sliding scale. Also, don't be shy about exploring whether you are eligible for a publicly funded medical insurance program. Every state provides medical coverage for its citizens who cannot afford to pay for private insurance, through a program that is called Medicaid in most states. The eligibility criteria vary tremendously from state to state, so you'll need to do a bit of research to see if you qualify. Your state's Department of Health Web site is a good place to start. Sometimes, you can even download application forms from the Web and jump-start the application process.

Should you apply for disability? The short answer is *not except as a last resort* and certainly not until you've had a thorough discussion with your therapist and other trusted advisers. Stopping work and losing the structure that it provides will lead to a tremendous vacuum in your life. The rhythms of the workday and workweek are tremendous organizing forces in our lives, and we give them up at our peril.

Acceptance and Committing to Getting Better

Remember that the most important member of your treatment team is you. If you don't make the commitment to be a contributing member of the team, treatment will not be effective, and improvement in symptoms and functioning will be as elusive for you as ever. Borderline personality disorder is not a problem that a professional can "fix" in you; successful treatment will require you to work very hard over a prolonged period, certainly many months, and often for several years.

It requires you to make a big commitment of time, money, and most of all, tremendous psychological effort.

The first step in making this commitment is acceptance. You have probably heard of the twelve steps that are the basis for several programs for recovery. These programs work from the principle that the person who wants to change needs to start on a journey toward health that moves from one step to the next. The first step is always the hardest to achieve: *I have acknowledged that I am powerless over (in this case, borderline personality disorder) and that my life has become unmanageable.* Unless you have achieved this step, recovery will remain out of reach.

Admitting that one is powerless over something is difficult to do but is utterly necessary for successful treatment for this problem. It means not making excuses or setting conditions or limits on doing what you need to do to get better.

This is important for us to emphasize because comprehensive treatment programs for borderline personality disorder are usually highly structured and intensive, with lots of confining rules and regulations. These will be about things like how many missed therapy appointments will be acceptable, mandatory attendance at groups for specified periods, and strict limits on how many phone calls to your therapist are permitted (and when). During the sessions of treatment addressing self-destructive behaviors, one of these conditions may include not discussing any trauma history for a set time because of the destabilizing effect it would have. Programs make these rules because they provide the structure needed for treatment to work. Time spent discussing whether a missed appointment was for a good reason or not, for example, is time taken away from what you need to be working on.

"I'll go to a skills-building group for three months, but I won't go for six; I don't see why that should be a requirement of the program" just won't work. Your life has become unmanageable, remember? So why are you trying to manage your treatment? You may as well not go at all; you're not ready.

All psychological treatment, at its core, is about learning how to live life differently, and it means developing new ways of thinking about yourself, about others in your life, and about the world around you. That means moving away from familiar ways of thinking and behaving. Even the most self-destructive behaviors can have a seductive appeal because of their familiarity—and that means they are difficult to give up. A principle of psychology is that people behave the way they do because on some level and in some fashion, that way of behaving *works* for them. Even the most self-destructive behaviors accomplish something, such as temporary relief from uncomfortable feelings, for example, and in a predictable way. Giving up these familiar coping mechanisms and relying on strangers, that is, therapists, and the ways of acting that they recommend, is not easy. Acceptance, however, makes it possible.

Treatment for the borderline personality diagnosis emphasizes acceptance from the beginning. *Mindfulness* is a mantra of these approaches, the awareness and acceptance of what *is*, right now, *as* it is, not as it "should" be, or as you would like it to be. Protesting that your treatment program's rules aren't reasonable, or aren't fair, or that they ask too much of you means you haven't achieved that first step. Move away from anger, accept how scary a prospect relinquishing so much control is for you—but do what needs to be done.

The Role of Hospitalization

Psychiatric hospitalization is often both frightening and comforting for persons who have borderline personality disorder, frightening because it is in many ways the ultimate relinquishing of control over self-determination. In the hospital, someone else determines when it's time to eat and sleep; there's often a lock on the entrance to the unit; visiting times and visitors are limited; and there are what seem like a thousand other limitations and restrictions. But the hospital is also a comforting prospect because someone else is in charge of *everything*, when you eat and sleep, and so forth. It's undeniably tempting to go someplace where you don't have to make any decisions about anything at all. The issue of hospitalization in many ways embodies one of the *dialectics* that characterize treatments for this problem, for it at once requires relinquishing control over many things to gain control over others.

Research has attempted to answer the question of whether psychiatric hospitalization is helpful in the long run for persons who have borderline personality disorder. There's no convincing evidence that it is—or that it isn't. Some facts, however, are clear. Psychiatric hospitalization provides a safe environment where people can be protected from self-destructive actions. But hospitalization is clearly not necessary for individuals to learn how to get control over self-destructive behaviors; ample research proves that outpatient treatment does that quite effectively. Some have argued that hospitalization is always harmful for individuals who have borderline personality disorder, that putting them in an environment where others are responsible for keeping them safe effectively prevents them from practicing the coping skills that they must master for themselves, or worse, that it sends the message that they won't be able to, or that treatment won't be effective. This can lead to ever more desperate attempts to cope—usually by using the same maladaptive behaviors and ways of communicating that may have triggered hospitalization in the first place—a phenomenon that has been called *regression*.

Like any other medical treatment, psychiatric hospitalization has risks and benefits and will be most effective when the patient and the treatment team have discussed both sides of this equation and pursue this course with concrete goals in mind: "What is the purpose of hospitalization *now*, for *me*?" "How will my treatment team and I know when that purpose has been achieved?" and just as important, "What should happen if satisfactory progress toward this goal is not being achieved in the hospital?" Other questions: "What are the negative consequences of hospitalization on my life?" (If your answer is, "I can't think of any," then you're not thinking hard enough.) "What should happen *after* hospitalization?" And after discharge from the hospital, "Could this hospitalization have been prevented?" and "What will decrease the chances of needing another hospitalization in the future?" Collaboratively developed answers to all these questions will greatly enhance the probability that hospitalization will be useful.

The Costs of Addiction

Nothing torpedoes psychiatric treatment as effectively as a substance abuse problem that has remained unaddressed. It's not even possible to provide an accurate psychiatric diagnosis if cycles of craving and seeking out substances, intoxication, withdrawal, and all the problems associated with addiction are clouding the picture (and remember what we said earlier about, "Diagnosis, diagnosis, diagnosis"). Alcohol, pills, and other substances all interfere with the brain's regulatory functioning. Persons who regularly use substances go through periods of depression, are more impulsive and lose control of their feelings more easily, experience disruptions in sleeping patterns and appetite, and lose interest in their usual pursuits as their energies become more and more centered on their substance use. It's not difficult to see how all these symptoms overlap with those of borderline personality disorder, as well as with mood disorders, making a correct psychiatric diagnosis virtually impossible.

People who are troubled by substance abuse problems in addition to other psychiatric problems like a mood disorder or BPD often convince themselves that their substance abuse is only a secondary problem, that their *other* problem is the true cause of their addiction, and that the addiction will disappear when their *other* problems are effectively treated. This is simply not true. Remember that addiction is a behavioral problem and that behaviors need to be interrupted, unlearned, and replaced by other, more healthy ways of behaving. A person who has a psychiatric illness and an addiction has *two* problems, *both* of which need to be addressed with the appropriate treatment. Treating either one will not make the other one go away. In fact, treating only one effectively will not be possible because each problem interferes with the treatment of the other.

Regular use of intoxicating substances chemically alters the brain in ways that interfere with the effectiveness of medications. An untreated mood disorder makes recovery from substance abuse nearly impossible. The terrible misery of depression or the loss of inhibitions that characterize the highs of bipolar disorder make it nearly impossible not to give into the temptation to assuage bad feelings or intensify good ones with intoxicants. Remember that persons who have BPD are impaired in their ability to regulate their feelings and self-soothe. If alcohol or pills have become a mainstay for you in achieving this modulation and soothing, you will not be able to learn how to accomplish these functions on your own.

It is absolutely imperative that you be accurate in reporting *exactly* what your substance use is to your treatment team. How much alcohol do you use and how often? The National Institute on Alcohol Abuse and Alcoholism considers four or more alcoholic drinks on one occasion in women and five or more drinks in men to indicate problem drinking (the NIAAA has several excellent self-assessment tools on their Web site: www.niaaa.nih.gov). If you are taking more pain pills or more antianxiety or sleep medications than your doctor prescribes, you likely have a problem. If you are buying pills "on the street," then you definitely have a problem.

One of us gives a lecture on the treatment of depression to medical students and psychiatric residents; on the summary slide in that lecture is this statement: "Patients who are abusing substances will not get better no matter what you do." In the landmark study of persons with borderline personality disorder carried out over ten years at McLean Hospital, the factor that was most associated with failure to recover from BPD symptoms and problems was an ongoing substance abuse problem.[2]

Treatment of severe substance abuse problems is also a specialized endeavor requiring professionals with specialized knowledge and experience. How does one know when such a professional is needed? Simply stated, when treatment as usual has not resulted in cessation of substance use. Alcohol and most of the prescription medications that individuals misuse cause physiological or physical addiction. This means that cutting down or suddenly stopping increases the risks of physical withdrawal symptoms. These not only are intensely uncomfortable but can be medically dangerous. Untreated alcohol withdrawal has a significant mortality rate. This is another reason it is important to be completely honest in reporting exactly what your substance use is to your treatment team so that detoxification can be safely carried out.

Remember that recovery from substance abuse is a process, not an event; it is often characterized by remissions and relapses. Don't get discouraged by setbacks. Have you seen those bumper stickers that read "One day at a time"? That is one of the mottos of Alcoholics Anonymous and an approach to recovery that will not steer you wrong.

Looking for Happiness in All the Wrong Places

Psychiatric treatment cannot make you happy. Sigmund Freud, in his *Studies on Hysteria,* talked about psychoanalysis being successful even if it only succeeded in replacing "neurotic misery" with "common unhappiness." Psychiatric treatment can help remove obstacles on your journey toward happiness, but a psychiatrist or psychotherapist cannot reveal to you the meaning of life, or tell you why *your* life is worth living. We are experts in the treatment of psychiatric disorders, not philosophers or theologians (or at least, that's not what we're trained in). Treatment for borderline personality disorder can help you learn how to cope with setbacks and disappointments better, negotiate relationships more successfully, rein in impulsiveness, make peace with a traumatic past and put it behind you, and many other important skills and lessons. Medication can relieve crippling depression or help check manic excesses. But your happiness is your responsibility, just as it is for everyone else.

We all find meaning and value in our relationships, work, spiritual values, artistic expression, and a thousand other aspects of life that differ enormously from one person to the next. The search for meaning and happiness cannot be restricted to the psychiatrist's or therapist's office or to the meeting room of a support group or group therapy. If you limit your searching to these rooms, then you are indeed looking for happiness in all the wrong places.

WE HOPE YOU ARE NOT DISCOURAGED after reading this chapter. We can understand why you might be. We've been telling you some potentially discouraging things: the diagnosis of the various problems associated with borderline personality is not easy to get right; treatment is complex, potentially expensive, and usually takes many months before it begins to pay off; and worst of all, successful treatment doesn't guarantee happiness.

But you shouldn't be discouraged. We've laid out some tough facts, buttressed by research and by experience, but only so that you know what you're up against and so that you *won't* get discouraged by how difficult getting better might be for you. Remember that borderline personality disorder is now thought of as a *good* prognosis diagnosis—don't let the challenges of getting better make you lose sight of that vital fact.

It took a while as I'd pretty much reached the bottom rung, but life is good for me now. I'm almost 15 years on and haven't purposefully injured myself in that time. I've had a number of jobs, got myself a career, a Ph.D. and some good friends. It's taken me a long while to pick up from where I left off at 9 years old but I think I'm there now, happy, settled and coping again.[3]

I did it—I am no longer a patient. I completed my degree, and am managing to work full-time. I no longer consider myself to have a diagnosis of borderline personality disorder. I have none of the symptoms and when I look around at other people I don't seem to be any different from anyone else. The only time I feel different is when I recognize that my journey to this point in my life has been a lot more complicated than many people I come into contact with. However, when I look around I also see myself handling situations more competently than many other people. I have gained in strength and resilience as a result of my experience of handling such intense emotions, which means that I am not easily overwhelmed by life's challenges. I'm not perfect though. I still have bad days, but talking to friends, so do most people. I really am no different. I no longer have thoughts of self-harm. My moods are more recognizable as normal, and my sense of self is much stronger and doesn't fragment anymore. In addition, I am more open, and able to recognize, contain and talk about my emotions. I can also manage friendships and intimate relationships. The only thing that is remotely borderline personality disordered about me now is that I can still remember how it felt to be that way—but it is just a memory.[3]

The motto of the university where both of us trained and now work is *Veritas vos Liberabit*, which translates to "The truth shall set you free." This is a variation on another saying you've probably heard: "Knowledge is power."

Truth and knowledge can make anything possible.

CHAPTER 15

For Parents, Partners, Friends, and Co-workers

Trying to help someone who has borderline personality disorder can be intensely frustrating and heartbreaking. Even the most patient and caring efforts to help might seem not only fruitless and unhelpful, but might actually make things worse. Throughout this book, we have given examples of how the various problems of persons with this diagnosis can feed on each other, setting up vicious cycles of crises that spiral out of control.

Perhaps more than with any other psychiatric problem, borderline personality disorder causes intense suffering not only for the person who has it, but for everyone who is close to that person. The daily stress and strain of living with a person who has this diagnosis is intense and pervasive. Family life seems to lurch relentlessly from crisis to crisis; family members are continuously reeling from emergencies, barely recovered from one before the next materializes.

We hope that having read much of this book, you have a better understanding of what this disorder is. This is the first step in learning how to help, and just as important, how to cope.

Our message throughout this book is that borderline personality disorder is best understood as a result of a multifaceted interaction of biology, temperament, and environment that results in a damaged sense of identity, an inability to modulate emotions, and a range of dysfunctional and self-destructive coping behaviors. We'll emphasize again that "personality" is only one piece of the equation, and that to call this set of problems simply a "personality disorder" is really quite inaccurate and inadequate. This unfortunate nomenclature means that many family members, on first hearing the diagnosis, can easily fall into one of several traps.

One trap is that simply saying someone has a "personality" problem is in many ways an indictment of her as a person. The message it gives is that she is to blame for all her problems and completely responsible for the unhappiness of those around her, and it's all because of *who she is*. The conclusion that one can logically draw from this is that pointing out her "character flaws" to her in the spirit of constructive criticism will help her change. But these individuals have great difficulty reacting positively to even the most well-intentioned criticism, especially if it is made in the midst of a crisis. Remember that one of the core features of this disorder is that the affected individual already feels that she is damaged, defective, bad—often irredeemably, hopelessly so. Criticism is often experienced as piercingly painful.

Criticism and its close relative, blaming, usually make people defensive and angry. An emotionally stable person, confident and secure in her image of herself as a reasonable, basically decent person, may be able to step back, objectively self-reflect on criticism, and see room for improvement in herself. When the person who has borderline personality disorder tries to "take a step back," however, she's confronted with a bottomless abyss of emptiness. With her damaged sense of self, being in the wrong means confronting her irreparable defectiveness. Arguments about who's right and who's wrong become literally life and death struggles. These individuals frequently cut themselves or make a suicide attempt after arguments with important persons in their lives.

Another trap set up by the term "personality disorder" is the implication that it can't be fixed, leading to a feeling of hopelessness or grim resignation that things will never change. Indeed, in chapters 2 and 5, where we discussed personality in detail, we repeatedly used the term *enduring* to describe it. There are two things to remember, though. First, "enduring" doesn't mean "permanent." Personality does change, albeit sometimes at what might seem like glacial speed; people can and do mature and, as they do so, learn to identify, take ownership of, and manage the extremes of their inborn temperament. Second, we want to emphasize once more that "borderline personality disorder" is much more than personality; it is also a mode of communicating and inter-acting and a set of dysfunctional and frightening behaviors—all prob-lems that are extremely amenable to treatment.

Several of our colleagues at Johns Hopkins are fond of saying, "*Do*, the feelings will come later." Interrupting dysfunctional behaviors and learning new coping and communication skills are cornerstones of successful treatment for this problem. And indeed, the feelings do "come later," as success in managing emotional over-reactions and the elimination of self-destructive behaviors gradually help the person's damaged sense of self heal.

We should also remind you that many of these individuals, in ad-dition to the problems we have just been discussing, have a treatable mood disorder. Persons who are in the grip of major depression or who are being constantly pummeled by the mood instability of a bipolar dis-order are quite incapable of learning new skills or interrupting problem behaviors. Treatment of these illnesses with the appropriate medica-tion can dramatically benefit these persons and accelerate progress in addressing their other issues. But this can be a trap, too. Family mem-bers can pin too much hope on medication (as can patients, their psy-chotherapists, and, yes, psychiatrists, too) and be tempted to put off or even think they can skip doing the hard work that must be done to ad-dress the other issues faced by families affected by this diagnosis.

Borderline personality disorder is a treatable condition that has what might even be described as an unusually good prognosis com-pared with many other psychiatric conditions; but defeating it requires a lot of work, a skilled treatment team, and most of all, perseverance, acceptance, and optimism.

Getting Someone into Treatment

Some of the most difficult conversations mental health profession-als have with family members of persons who have mental illness are those with parents, partners, or adult children pleading for help in get-ting a seriously ill relative into treatment—a relative who steadfastly professes, "I don't have a problem."

Some persons who have BPD and are not receiving treatment are not terribly impaired in many basic areas of life. Some go to work every day; many live independently—few signs of their severe problems may be visible to the outside world. At home, however, the angry outbursts, the heated arguments, the varied personal and family crises take an intolerable toll.

First, families must agree on who has the problem and needs to get treatment for it. Professionals who treat these patients learn to quickly recognize what has been called *splitting*. Splitting, in simple terms, is playing off one person against the other. A hospitalized patient will tell a nurse, "I can talk to you because *you* understand me. Dr. Jones doesn't listen like you do." If the nurse is inexperienced, she may find herself persuaded that Dr. Jones *doesn't* listen to the patient and find herself advocating for the patient to Dr . Jones, perhaps disagreeing with Dr. Jones about some aspect of the treatment plan. Suddenly, the patient's conflict has been transformed into conflict between nurse and doctor. The patient becomes like the eye of a hurricane, coolly unaffected by a conflict between others that starts swirling around him. You may know that the eye of a hurricane is the part of the hurricane where the atmospheric pressure is lowest. Splitting works the same way: pressure to change gets transferred from the patient to the people around him. Substitute "Mom" and "Dad" for "nurse" and "Dr. Jones" in this scenario and you can see how destructive this process can be.

The person who has BPD may persuade his mother that if only Dad would be more flexible, or more understanding, or more forgiving, things at home would be much better. The parents can start to criticize and blame each other for the turmoil at home. Or perhaps Dad simply throws up his hands and declares, "Leave me out of it!" and withdraws. In either case—and there are an infinite number of other such scenarios—everyone has become distracted from the real issue: the symptoms and need for treatment of the person who has BPD.

Splitting is theorized to be a basic element of the range of dysfunctional coping mechanisms of persons with this diagnosis, an outgrowth of the person's black-and-white, all-good or all-bad way of looking at the world. These individuals are not doing this consciously; rather, the behavior reflects how they see the world. They are seeking support and reassurance in every possible way from any source available; splitting is one inevitable result. The solution to splitting behaviors is communication: everyone needs to operate with the same set of information (this means no secrets, not ever, from anyone) and get on the same page as far as next steps.

Once other family members agree, communication with the person who has BPD about the need for psychological evaluation can begin. It should never begin, however, in the heat of an argument or other crisis. First, when people are angry, defensive, and trading blame, the process becomes one about who "wins" and who "loses" the argument, a setup for resentments. Also, making psychiatric treatment the focus of an argument can have the effect of equating treatment with punishment for bad behavior in the individual's mind, thus torpedoing the most basic requirement for effective psychological treatment: going into it with an open mind and a willingness to take advice and work to change.

Persons with the borderline diagnosis invariably go through periods of depression and intense mental anguish, and in those times, they may be much more willing to entertain the idea of mental health treatment to address their misery. Fortunately, most people have become much more accepting of the idea that severe depression is a treatable problem, and depressed persons invariably want to feel better. Suggesting a mental health evaluation to make a diagnosis, which is absolutely necessary for developing a successful treatment approach, has a much better chance of being accepted when it is offered as a course of action to make someone feel better.

Family members must be wary about making ultimatums about treatment, or worse, somehow tricking their loved one into a psychological evaluation. This frequently has the effect of steeling the patient's resolve *against* treatment. We frequently see patients brought less than willingly to an evaluation appointment that ends up being nothing more than a "Yes, you did! No I *didn't!*" session—in other words, a useless exercise for all involved.

In some circumstances, however, a person's refusal to seek treatment is not acceptable. If behaviors are putting her own safety or the safety of others at imminent risk, inaction is not an option, and some kind of intervention becomes necessary—whether the person welcomes intervention or not.

Hospitalization and Involuntary Treatment

Every community has laws to safeguard individuals who are unable to care for themselves. The most obvious example are laws allowing the removal of children from the care of parents who are abusing them. Another set of laws allows the treatment of individuals for psychiatric illnesses against their will in certain circumstances. One of the most difficult things a parent or partner might be called on to do for a family member who has a psychiatric illness is to initiate involuntary treatment or hospitalization for their loved one over her protests.

The laws governing involuntary psychiatric treatment are mostly state laws, so they vary from one state to another; in addition, local procedures often vary from community to community. This means that we can't provide a step-by-step procedure here, only general principles.

Law and legal procedures governing the provision of psychiatric treatment (or any kind of medical treatment for that matter) against a person's stated wishes are based on the knowledge that an individual whose judgment is clouded by the symptoms of an illness often does not make the same decisions about his treatment that he would make otherwise. The delirious motor vehicle accident victim who has suffered massive blood loss may moan "I want to go home" as he loses consciousness on the gurney, but the emergency department team will ignore such a statement and proceed to do what's necessary to save the person's life. It is presumed that if the person were alert and thinking clearly and understood the implications of "going home," he would not make such a request. No one would ask a screaming toddler for written permission for a needed blood test. Similar principles underlie psychiatric commitment law: treatment is given to persons against their will if clouded judgment prevents them from making good decisions about their treatment.

Fortunately, these laws also have safeguards built in to prevent confinement in a psychiatric hospital for the wrong reasons. Decades ago, it was easy to invoke commitment law, which often required only the signature of a relative or family physician to hospitalize a person for weeks or months, even years. People were hospitalized for all kinds of bogus reasons, and serious abuses of individual rights occurred. Laws became much stricter in the 1960s and 1970s to prevent these abuses. The main change was the addition of *dangerousness* as a commitment criterion. Unless an individual's behavior endangers himself (usually meaning suicidal behavior) or others, he cannot be committed for involuntary psychiatric treatment.

Requests or petitions for psychiatric hospitalization do not necessarily mean that the person who is alleged to be psychiatrically ill will be hospitalized. Relatives cannot simply sign a person into a facility; only a doctor can admit someone to a hospital. (In Maryland, where we practice, involuntary commitment actually requires that two physicians, or a physician and a psychologist, independently agree that the person requires an admission.) A parent's request for her child's admission or involuntary commitment usually allows the child to be transported to an emergency department of a hospital, where a physician will make a decision about hospitalization. The person may be released if he does not meet legal criteria for involuntary commitment.

Involuntary commitment is a serious legal procedure in which an individual is confined against his will and temporarily loses some of his rights of self-determination. For this reason the law and the courts take involuntary psychiatric treatment very seriously, and many safeguards against abuses are built into the procedures. The person requesting an involuntary commitment must usually appear in person at the local courthouse or police station to give information and, in some jurisdictions, make a sworn statement before a judge or magistrate. This person is asked to provide specific and detailed information about behaviors, which is often frustrating for those trying to get help for their loved one. They may feel that being asked a lot of questions is uncaring, or that someone is questioning their judgment or their motives. It's important to remember that when individuals could be confined to psychiatric hospitals simply because a relative or doctor "thought it was best" for them, there were significant abuses of civil rights. The issuing magistrate or judge's serious attention to documenting the facts and to close questioning of the need for involuntary treatment of adults means that the system is working.

The definition, or perhaps more accurately the legal interpretation, of what *dangerousness* means varies tremendously from one jurisdiction to another. Personal testimony by someone who actually heard a relative threaten to take his life may be required. Threats to hurt someone else also qualify. In other areas, simply the "likelihood" that the person would harm himself or another person if untreated is the language used in the law. Self-mutilation, for the most part, is taken at face value as dangerous behavior. Some states also provide for involuntary commitment of substance-abusing persons for treatment of their addiction.

There is some form of judicial review (a *commitment hearing*) at some point (usually a few days after hospitalization), where a judge or hearing officer determines that the admission procedure was done properly and legally. Although this is a legal proceeding, it is not a big courtroom scene. Usually a conference room in the hospital is used, only a few people are present, and the proceedings are kept confidential (not a matter of public record). The patient is allowed legal representation; an attorney will be appointed to represent the patient if he does not have one. In some jurisdictions, if the patient is a minor, even when both parents and child agree to hospitalization, a similar hearing occurs to safeguard the rights of the minor.

Involuntary commitment for psychiatric treatment does not affect a person's other legal rights. Wills or other legal instruments he has executed are not invalidated, and patients do not become legally "incompetent" in other areas. Hospitalization and treatment are the only issues addressed in commitment hearings.

We are aware that this topic is frightening; it might seem that a person's liberty and the right of self-determination can be taken away all too easily. At the risk of sounding glib, however, we want to reassure you that involuntary commitment of an individual is *not* a quick and easy procedure. On the contrary, most people are surprised at how difficult it is to invoke these laws, how many safeguards are built into the procedures, and how seriously the strict interpretation of the laws is taken by everyone involved. These laws have been carefully written in the interest of helping, not simply confining, people with severe psychiatric illnesses.

Safety Issues

Never forget that psychiatric disorders can occasionally precipitate truly dangerous behavior. The dark specter of suicidal violence haunts those with serious depression, and the rageful irritability of persons who have BPD can lead to frightening assaultiveness. Gruesome and dangerous self-mutilation is unfortunately common in persons who have this diagnosis.

Violence is often a difficult subject for people to deal with because the idea is deeply embedded in us from an early age that violence is primitive and uncivilized and represents a kind of failure or breakdown in character. Of course we recognize that the person in the grip of psychiatric illness is not violent because of some personal failing, and perhaps because of this, there is sometimes a hesitation to admit the need for a proper response to a situation that is getting out of control, when there is some threat of violence, toward self or others.

Although family members cannot and should not be expected to take the place of psychiatric professionals in evaluating risk for self-harm, it is important to have some familiarity with the issue. As we've already mentioned, persons who self-harm are often intensely ashamed of these behaviors. Many are ashamed about having suicidal thoughts as well. These individuals may hint about "feeling desperate," or about not being able to "go on," but they may not verbalize actual self-destructive thoughts. It's important not to ignore these statements but to clarify them. Don't be afraid to ask, "Are you having thoughts of hurting yourself?" if you suspect your relative may be. People are oftentimes relieved to be able to talk about these feelings and get them out in the open where they can be dealt with, but they may need permission and support to do so. When the person feels invisible or ignored or that her pain is being minimized, these behaviors can escalate in the attempt to get someone to take her seriously so that she is not alone with what she experiences as literally intolerable distress. Sometimes, if the person is able to acknowledge the urge to harm herself, the permission to say so out loud may reduce the intensity of what she is experiencing, especially if all this occurs within the context of a family crisis plan that has been previously developed.

Another factor that increases risk of all self-harming behaviors is substance abuse, especially alcohol abuse. Alcohol not only worsens mood; it lowers inhibitions. People will do things when they are drunk that they wouldn't do otherwise. Increased use of alcohol increases the risk of suicidal behaviors and is definitely a worrisome development that needs to be confronted and acted on.

The development of serious suicidal risk calls for action, as does the risk of violence toward others. Friends and family members should not hesitate to call for police help if they feel threatened.

Have an emergency plan and be prepared to use it. This planning and information gathering about procedures is immensely important. The last thing you want to do is improvise and guess in the midst of an emergency because of an information vacuum. Don't hesitate to invoke involuntary commitment procedures if you are really worried and the person is not cooperating with the need for evaluation.

"What will the neighbors think?" should not be a worry where safety issues are concerned. If the situation is becoming dangerous, don't call the psychiatrist's office or the local emergency room, as the advice you get there will simply be a variation on this theme: dial 911. EMTs and police officers are accustomed to dealing with psychiatrically ill individuals. They know safe physical restraint techniques, and they will be familiar with psychiatric emergency services in the community. They will have the same goals you will in the situation: transporting the person quickly and safely to the appropriate health care facility so that she can receive proper treatment.

Recognizing and Addressing Abusive Behaviors

Parents and partners often need help with handling their loved one's abusive behaviors toward them. In preparation for writing this chapter, to learn more about what family members wanted and needed, we looked at several online resources offering support for family members of persons who have borderline personality disorder. It quickly became apparent, however, that we had little to learn there. First, the questions and needs we found were no different from those we had encountered in the families of our own patients, but more important, many of these forums were filled with messages from family members who were simply venting their frustration. And although this kind of release has its place—at least briefly—it really doesn't do anyone much good in the long run.

Why? Because frequently, venting about problems becomes a substitute for, rather than a prelude to, actually *doing* something, taking useful action. Some of these unfortunate family members even seemed to take a perverse pride in telling their tales of abuse, seemingly trying to outdo each other by describing what "my BP did to me today." In these families, the person who had BPD had indeed become the "eye of the hurricane" that we discussed, with the family's life being reduced to wreckage around her. Venting about it may garner kind and sympathetic words, but what these family members really need is someone to teach them how to set limits on and impose consequences for the abusive behaviors of their relative.

Psychiatric illness may be an explanation for a person's emotionally and perhaps even physically abusive behaviors toward family members, but it is not an excuse. Remember the crucial difference between psychiatric illness, what the person *has*, and problem behaviors, what the person *does*. Although no one is to blame for having a psychiatric illness or for having extremes of personality, everyone is responsible for what they *do*. As we have emphasized elsewhere in this book, maladaptive behaviors are quite amenable to proper treatment, making it even more important not to explain them away.

Tolerating abusive behaviors or shielding persons with psychiatric problems from the appropriate consequences of illegal acts sends them the message that continuing the behaviors is acceptable. Just calling a handyman to repair the hole in the wall that the person made in a moment of rage after yet another "please don't do this again" speech has only the minutest chance of preventing a recurrence. Pleading with a neighbor not to press charges after he's been assaulted or his property has been vandalized because "after all, she *is* mentally ill," may be precisely the *worst* course of action to help the person who has BPD. What to do instead? There are never easy answers to that question. "What to do" needs to be developed on an ongoing basis; the best process for doing so will involve consultation with a professional who is trained and experienced in helping manage these situations.

As we discussed in the section on dialectical behavioral therapy, family sessions are sometimes built into this treatment technique. Family therapy will definitely be included in DBT for adolescent patients. For adults, it is more often an adjunctive treatment, frequently short term and time limited. Seeing a family therapist or couples' counselor who is not the patient's individual therapist is often the most effective means of addressing these issues. If the person who has BPD is refusing treatment, then family members may need to arrange to get psychological treatment for themselves alone.

The bottom line here is that persons with this diagnosis are profoundly troubled in their relationships and impaired in their ability to negotiate the inevitable give-and-take of family life; they tend to project their emotional pain outward onto those around them, whom they blame for their difficulties. Tantrums, manipulation, and emotional blackmail may be ways of dealing with emotional pain for them. Logical persuasion, attempts to understand and compromise, kindness, constructive criticism, and all the other strategies for solving relationship problems that are usually effective are often quite ineffective in dealing with the conflicts that repeatedly arise with these individuals. Instead, special techniques are needed, and family members almost always need instruction, coaching, and support to master them.

These techniques and strategies are so varied and individualized that it would be foolish and inadequate for us to attempt much detail here. However, laying out a few general principles may be helpful to you.

One principle is that nothing useful is ever accomplished during an argument. When does a discussion become an argument? The line may be hard to define, but everyone knows when they've crossed it. When *you* feel like you're arguing, then that line has been crossed—no matter what the opinion of the others in the room. At that point, one should declare unilateral cessation of combat operations and withdraw. "I'm too upset to continue talking about this anymore, so we are not going to solve this issue now. We can discuss it later when I'm not feeling angry." And that is the end of the discussion/argument. Change the subject, walk out of the room if necessary, but make it clear that it's over for now. When you are angry and upset, you are not entirely in control and are more likely to say negative things, or make promises or threats that you may later regret.

Another principle is that everyone is entitled to his feelings and responsible for his behavior. Just as feeling like you're arguing means you are, if you are feeling harassed, then someone is harassing you. If you feel abused, then someone is abusing you. And if someone is harassing or abusing you, he needs to be informed of it, told to stop, and if necessary, reminded of the consequences of not stopping.

One aspect of most personality disorders is that the person has great difficulty accurately gauging the emotions and feelings of others. We have had patients who have antisocial personality disorder and are facing criminal charges after making threats tell us something along the lines of, "She shouldn't have been scared of me; she should know that I didn't really mean it." We tell these patients that if someone is frightened of you, *then you have frightened that person,* and there are consequences for doing so. This principle bears repeating: *everyone is entitled to his feelings and is responsible for his behaviors.*

Another principle that stems from this one is the importance of following through on consequences. Consequences are best framed as, "If X, then Y" statements. "I will help you out with your rent this time, but if you miss another payment, then I will not pay it for you again, and you cannot move back home." Notice that "If X, then Y" is not open to interpretation. Trouble is ahead if instead of this simplicity, the statement is more complicated, for example, "If X, then Y, unless, of course, Z, or possibly Q." When too much judgment, or, worst of all, assessment of feelings go into the algorithm, consequences are bound to be ineffective. Behavioral psychologists talk about "extinguishing" an unwanted behavior in an animal (or a person) and know that it is extremely difficult to extinguish a behavior unless negative reinforcement is delivered consistently and predictably, every single time the behavior occurs. Omitting the negative reinforcement, or, in this case, not following through on the promised consequences even once, will result in the behavior being even more difficult to extinguish going forward.

Following through on consequences can be difficult. Individuals who have BPD sometimes engage in a sort of hostage taking to prevent it, by threatening to harm themselves to force others to give in. We are often told by families that implementing negative consequences is "impossible . . . if I take away her cell phone, she'll kill herself!" These sorts of traps eliminate the threat of negative consequences for the person by implying worse, unacceptably negative consequences for the family. Dealing with these situations is never easy—it is one of the reasons that DBT therapists need their own support groups to do this work. As we stated above, these matters are so individualized that attempting to lay out a one-size-fits-all strategy would be not only futile but misleading. The participation of an experienced mental health professional is critical in establishing a plan for how to react to these situations. If the person who has BPD will not get into her own therapy, for whatever reason, family therapy or individual therapy for the parent or spouse can be incredibly helpful.

Another important rule, one that is quite self-explanatory, is that everyone needs to *say what they mean, and mean what they say*. This is another aspect of holding everyone accountable for their actions.

The final principle we'll lay out for parents and partners is that you can decide that enough is enough; in fact, *only* you can decide when that line has been crossed. It is up to you to determine when your situation has become so intolerable and irretrievable, at least temporarily, that you need to unilaterally sever a relationship. Others can give you advice and counsel, but you need no one's permission. Seek advice about how to proceed; this may be as simple as asking your phone company how to block incoming calls from a particular phone number, or as complicated as consulting an attorney to draw up legal separation papers. But you are entitled to decide that your physical, psychological, or financial well-being is in jeopardy and that self-protection is necessary and then take the appropriate actions.

Borderline Personality Disorder in the Workplace

Because borderline personality disorder is almost defined by difficult interpersonal relationships, it should not be surprising that a person with this diagnosis has the potential to be an extremely disruptive influence in the workplace. It has been estimated that about half of persons diagnosed with borderline personality disorder have severe impairments in their ability to remain employed.[1] Even individuals with the diagnosis who can function in other settings can be undone by the need to cooperate, collaborate, and otherwise productively interact with co-workers in a work environment, where interpersonal dealings are expected to remain professional. Many people with this diagnosis simply can't muster the ability to remain cool and collected under these demands.

Their co-workers experience people with borderline symptoms simply as difficult and judge them to be "manipulative" or "immature." The emotional instability inherent in the disorder results in extreme and rapid changes in emotions in response to good news or bad. Co-workers will find themselves cleaning up mistakes, dealing with passive-aggressive behaviors, constantly worrying about retaliation, or just getting fed up with all the drama these persons seem to continually activate.

Managers with the diagnosis will typically interpret interpersonal approval as more important than productivity and will invite subordinates to compete for their attention, giving special attention to favored ones regardless of their productivity.

Co-workers may sense that what is wrong with their colleague involves a psychiatric problem, but the diagnosis of borderline personality disorder is often unfamiliar. "Maybe she has multiple personalities," they may think; or "He must be bipolar." Problematic behaviors come from a very deep distress within people who have borderline personality disorder. Although co-workers often feel angry about or resentful of these behaviors, the people in question are certainly not having fun but are suffering deeply and expressing this suffering through behavior that is often destructive, both to others and to themselves.

What if your employee has these characteristics? Your co-worker? Your boss? Much of the advice given elsewhere in this book, including trying to persuade the person to get into treatment, isn't appropriate in the workplace. Managers may try ignoring the problem and attempt to work around it by giving extra tasks and responsibility to other employees—a perfect recipe for demoralization and conflict in the workplace. Others collect enough evidence of workplace misbehavior to justify firing the employee and in that way eliminate the workplace problem—but to many, this approach seems cruel and uncaring, and for the employee, it certainly reinforces the negative cognitions and abandonment that drive borderline behaviors in the first place.

An entire field of study has sprung up within the institutional psychology literature that specifically focuses on *counterproductive workplace behavior* (CWB). Such behavior is defined as "any intentional behavior on the part of an organization member viewed by the organization as contrary to its legitimate interests."[2] Generally, the recommendations of specialists in this field center on decreasing the "personal" in interpersonal relationships in the workplace.

Managing an Employee Who Has BPD

Managers may supervise an employee who seems to be arguing with them constantly, often seemingly just for the sake of arguing. They may notice an employee who is harshly critical of the workplace, the management, or another employee around peers and subordinates but who quickly disavows his comments when the manager asks about them. An employee with BPD may trigger conflicts in the workplace by playing one person against another in some way. The effect of these problems on the manager can be profound. Emotionally, the manager may feel defeated and drained. Practically, dealing with these issues takes away valuable time that could be put to better use. Managers may find various techniques helpful in managing these employees.

Setting clear boundaries and expectations for productivity, and providing regular feedback using objective measures, lays a foundation. Unfortunately, one of the core features of borderline personality disorder, the damaged sense of identity, means that even completely fair, objective, and appropriate workplace limits (such as not dating co-workers) are frequently experienced as personal and punitive by persons who have BPD.

Because the problems are interpersonal, rather than occupational, a good strategy is to separate these two types of relationships. Most people with BPD will (often without realizing it) have great difficulty managing this divide—they highly prioritize the interpersonal aspects of relationships and have difficulty recognizing the occupational ones. Consequently, they frequently experience occupational limits as interpersonal rejection and react accordingly. Interpersonal support, combined with firm and objective occupational goals and limits, can be an excellent combination. The strategy may include weekly progress meetings, dividing up large tasks into smaller constituent ones (each of which must be turned in to the manager for supervision), and keeping detailed logs of the employee's time at work. Taking the time to explain (and repeat as necessary) the difference between occupational and interpersonal expectations can actually help the person not only in the workplace but also in his life beyond work. Emphasizing that picking another person for a particular task is not showing favoritism, but rather is making a decision based on the other employee's experience in this area, is a more understanding and effective approach than either (a) promising the next project to the employee or (b) refusing to explain at all.

Perhaps the worst thing the workplace manager can do is attempt to delve into the personal reasons for their BPD employee's workplace difficulties and become a confidante or counselor. Once broached, this boundary is not easily re-established, and the manager will find herself complicit and embroiled in her employee's conflicts rather than being able to serve, appropriately, as an objective problem solver. Employees need to be accountable for their workplace *behaviors*, and the compassionate manager needs to tell her employee to "do what he needs to do" to solve whatever personal problems he may have. Tolerating unacceptable behaviors gives the message that they are acceptable after all. Getting well and getting these behaviors under control are the responsibility of the person who has BPD and his professional caregivers, not of his boss or his colleagues.

Working with Someone Who Has BPD

Perhaps you are confronted with borderline traits in a co-worker, someone with whom you must collaborate to maintain a productive work environment. Because people who work together are effectively social peers, unaffected people often find themselves caught up in the unpredictable whirlwind that people who have BPD unknowingly create. A pervasive feeling that one must always "walk on eggshells" around a certain co-worker develops because the person who has BPD seems to switch moods in reaction to minor stimuli. People with this diagnosis typically have intense "hot and cold" interpersonal relationships that cause them to have difficulty working collaboratively on a consistent basis with everyone else. Because the person who has borderline disorder is unpredictable, co-workers may feel as if they are shouldering more of the work burden. They may feel that their hard effort goes unnoticed, as most of the attention in the workplace is taken up dealing with the employee who has BPD. And if co-workers try to set firm limits, their efforts can be met with resistance, anger, complaints, and occasionally what psychiatrists call an *extinction burst*, in which bad behavior actually increases before it begins to dissipate.

Individuals with BPD generally place more importance on interpersonal relationships than on workplace productivity. They may feel that as long as they are in a relationship with the right players, actual productivity is less important. As such, they may react to perceived interpersonal slights with retaliation or even sabotage. The best way to handle these situations is to discuss the problem with a trusted manager or superior. It then falls to that person to attend to the problem (as it should). Although an employee may be hesitant to take this step because it feels like "telling" on the co-worker, the alternative is to simply try to ignore the negative behaviors of one's colleague, which leads to resentment, anxiety, and an overall negative workplace experience.

Working for Someone Who Has BPD

Having a manager with borderline personality disorder can be highly anxiety provoking. The manager is usually responsible for not only supervising subordinates, but also for representing them to the senior management of the organization and mentoring them in their professional development. When one's workplace success depends more on an interpersonal relationship than on workplace performance, the workplace becomes highly competitive in unhealthy ways. Employees feel that they are always in a popularity contest, one for which they don't know the rules. The relationship is constantly in flux and unpredictable, due to the unpredictability of the emotions of those who have BPD. One person commented to us, "I never know who is going to walk into the office in the morning, the good [manager] or the mean [manager]." Her situation became so extreme that she saved multiple versions of her reports, because there were times when different text formatting could positively or negatively affect the "quality" of the report in the manager's eyes.

Properly navigating this situation can seem a daunting task, and at times it feels like walking a tightrope. If the employee tries to ignore the interpersonal struggles to "just get my work done and go home," the manager may feel rejected and retaliate against the employee. If, on the other hand, the employee tries to get in sync with the manager and prioritize their interpersonal relationship over productivity, he may find himself on a rocky road at best and unemployed at worst. If the manager's issues are truly getting in the way of a successful workplace environment, the best solution can be discussing the situation with other people. You may find that everyone has had similar experiences, and you and the others may be able to discuss these experiences with the manager's supervisor. Fundamentally, the manager is not performing her function and is probably not enjoying work any more than you are. Addressing the problem directly, rather than skirting the issue, will often help everyone be more satisfied and successful.

Getting Support

It's important that family members recognize their own need for support, encouragement, and understanding in dealing with this problem. Mental health professionals go home every day and leave their work of dealing with psychiatric illnesses behind, an option that parents and partners do not have. Individuals with this diagnosis are almost by definition some of the most frustrating and emotionally draining individuals to live with. The relentlessness and pervasiveness of their problems intrude into every aspect of home life, a source of severe stress in family relationships that strain them to the breaking point.

But a hard lesson is learning that no one can *force* an individual to take responsibility for her treatment. Unless the person makes the commitment to do so, no amount of love and support, sympathy and understanding, cajoling or even threatening can make someone take this step. Even those who understand this at some level can feel guilty, inadequate, and angry while dealing with this situation. These are normal feelings, and you should not be ashamed of the frustration and anger—get help with them.

Even when the person who has BPD does take responsibility and tries to stay well, relapses can occur. Family members might wonder what *they* did wrong. Did I put too much pressure on him? Could I have been more supportive? Why didn't I notice the symptoms coming on sooner and get him to the doctor? A hundred questions, a thousand "if only's." Another round of guilt, frustration, and anger.

On the other side of this issue is another question: How much understanding and support for the person who has borderline personality disorder might be too much? What's protective and what is overprotective? What actions constitute helping a sick person and what actions are helping a person to be sick? These are thorny questions that have no easy answers.

For all these reasons, it's vital that family members seek out support groups and organizations and consider getting counseling or therapy for themselves to deal with the stresses caused by these problems. Like many other illnesses, borderline personality disorder afflicts one but affects many in the family. It's important that *all* those affected get the help, support, and encouragement they need.

Epilogue

If the causes of borderline personality disorder could be summed up in a few sentences, they would read something like this:

Borderline personality disorder develops when a child born with extremes of temperament and a biologically rooted difficulty managing emotions encounters a mismatched childhood environment. This mismatch may be quite subtle or quite pathological but is experienced by the child as inconsistent and unpredictable, leading her to develop a damaged sense of self and the expectation that others will continue to be inconsistent, unpredictable, and ultimately unreliable and abandoning. This in turn causes profound emptiness and hopelessness to dominate her emotional life. To cope with her emotional extremes, and her desperate and painful unhappiness, she develops self-destructive coping behaviors like addictions, eating disorders, and self-mutilation. Frequently, these individuals also suffer from biologically based mental illnesses that exacerbate all their other problems and prevent behavioral and psychological treatments from helping them.

Well, that's more than few sentences, isn't it? But that is about the best we can do to distill this complicated disorder down to its essences. Notice that "essences" is plural here, to emphasize that there is no *one* essence or causative factor for this disorder.

Borderline personality disorder results from an interaction of genetic and other biological factors, inborn temperament, and childhood experiences and is usually complicated by the development of abnormal behaviors and psychiatric illnesses. All these factors require therapeutic attention, often by different professionals using different approaches. We have already quoted the old saying that, "There's always

Table E.1 Future needs and directions for borderline personality disorder

Increased public awareness is needed to decrease the stigma of borderline personality disorder, increase recognition of the disorder among therapists and physicians, and increase the availability of appropriate treatment.

Further research on the description, course, treatment, and epidemiology of mood disorders and anxiety disorders should also document the co-occurrence and effects of borderline personality disorder on patients with both conditions.

Psychiatric residency programs should be required to include training on borderline personality disorder.

Centers of excellence are needed to develop a new generation of borderline personality disorder researchers and clinicians.

Source: Adapted from J. Gunderson, "Borderline personality disorder: Ontogeny of a diagnosis," *American Journal of Psychiatry* 166 (2009): 530–39.

a simple answer to a complicated question, and it's always wrong." This is certainly true for borderline personality disorder. Successful treatments are available, and clinical research shows that most people will recover from this disorder. Although there are no shortcuts, *recovery*, not just remission or symptom control, unlike with many other psychiatric disorders, is an achievable goal for patients, their therapists and psychiatrists, and their family and friends. The journey may be long and arduous, but a new kind of life is a destination within reach.

Still, there are challenges and unmet needs, especially the need for wider availability of the new proven treatment approaches. Dr. John Gunderson, arguably one of the leading experts of the disorder in the twenty-first century, suggests that better treatment for patients includes promoting wider awareness of the disorder, among the general public and among professionals; investment in research and training on the disorder; and wider appreciation of the overlap between borderline personality disorder and other psychiatric illnesses (table E.1).

We intend for this book to be an optimistic resource for a psychiatric disorder that, for decades, was considered essentially untreatable. Those dark days are now over for good, and the future is increasingly bright. We want to leave you on this optimistic note.

In 2008, the United States House of Representatives unanimously passed House Resolution 1005 establishing the month of May as "Borderline Personality Disorder Awareness Month." The resolution stated that "despite its prevalence, enormous public health costs, and the devastating toll it takes on individuals, families, and communities, [borderline personality disorder] only recently has begun to command the attention it requires." The resolution calls it "essential to increase awareness of BPD among people suffering from this disorder, their families, mental health professionals, and the general public by promoting education, research, funding, early detection, and effective treatments." It is our sincere hope that this book contributes to the achievement of this lofty, but very attainable goal.

> *Courage does not always roar. Sometimes courage is a little voice at the end of the day that says "I'll try again tomorrow."*
> —Mary Anne Radmacher

APPENDIX A

Resources and Further Reading

ONLINE RESOURCES

National Education Alliance for Borderline Personality Disorder (NEA for BPD) www.borderlinepersonalitydisorder.com

Formed in 2001, this nonprofit advocacy and support organization was created specifically to educate the general public about borderline personality disorder. They hold educational conferences both locally and nationally. They also have their own twelve-week course for families, which focuses on education and skills training.

Behavioral Tech, LLC, Clinical Resource Directory
http://behavioraltech.org

This is Dr. Marsha Linehan's organization, which focuses on educating the public about and training professionals on dialectic behavioral therapy. This Web site contains mountains of information about borderline personality disorder and DBT. Therapists can find opportunities for information and training, and persons who have borderline personality disorder and their families will find resources as well. There is also a searchable database of clinicians in every state who have completed DBT training with Linehan's group.

National Alliance on Mental Illness (NAMI)
www.nami.org

Founded in 1979, NAMI strives to improve the lives of those suffering with mental illness. They have numerous locations throughout the USA and various support groups for patients and families. The borderline personality disorder section of NAMI's Web site is found by clicking on "Mental Illness."

National Institute of Mental Health (NIMH)

www.nimh.nih.gov/health/topics/borderline-personality-disorder

> The NIMH is primarily a government-funded research organization, but they have expanded their mission to include providing education and support on psychiatric conditions. The section on borderline personality disorder has educational information, tools to find providers in one's area, and links to more recent research and progress in the fight against borderline personality disorder.

Borderline Personality Disorder Resource Center

http://bpdresourcecenter.org

> This one-stop shop for all things related to BPD was created by Otto Kernberg, the creator of transference-focused psychotherapy. However, it strives to give unbiased representations of many therapeutic options for patients and their families. It also includes a large number of informational and preventive resources.

SUGGESTED READINGS

Other Conditions That Commonly Co-occur with Borderline Personality Disorder

Mondimore, F. M. 2006. *Bipolar Disorder: A Guide for Patients and Families,* 2nd ed. Baltimore: Johns Hopkins University Press.

> "Exhaustive, scientific, yet compassionate . . . An absolute gold mine for those with the disorder and their families: thorough, candid, and up-to-date advice, full of new possibilities for help."—*Kirkus Reviews*

> "I highly recommend it for patients and their family members and friends as an enlightened, pragmatic, and empathic resource for this very complex and challenging illness."—*Journal of Clinical Psychiatry*

Mondimore, F. M. 2006. *Depression, The Mood Disease,* 3rd ed. Baltimore: Johns Hopkins University Press.

> "If it seems a gloomy thought to explore the workings of mental doldrums, psychiatrist Mondimore makes this a safe trip, explaining in simple language how depression and manic-depression take effect and what victims can do about it."—*Publishers Weekly*

> "This is a reader friendly book on depression and mood disorders written primarily for patients and their families. It explains scientific and clinical facts at a patient level helping the patient get a better bearing on the nature of depression."—Doody's Review Service

Siegel, M., J. Brisman, and M. Weinshel. 2009. *Surviving an Eating Disorder: Strategies for Families and Friends*, 3rd ed. New York: HarperCollins.

"Well organized and extensive . . . The reasonable and practical suggestions provide numerous insights into helpful changes that can be tried by parents, spouses, friends and even the identified patient." —Vivian Meehan, President, National Association of Anorexia Nervosa and Related Disorders

Inspiration and Skills Building

De Mello, A. 1984. *The Song of the Bird*. New York: Image Press.

Anthony de Mello, a Jesuit priest, shares 124 stories from a variety of traditions to illustrate profound contemporary realities about our everyday concerns and our common spiritual quest.

Aitken, R. 1994. *Encouraging Words: Zen Buddhist Teachings for Western Students*. New York: Pantheon Books.

"*Encouraging Words* will appeal to both beginning and advanced lay Zen students who seek to integrate their spiritual practice into everyday life. Curious readers will be rewarded, too. Here is a teacher both wise and practical in equal measure."—*Honolulu Advertiser*

De Mello, A., and J. F. Stroud, eds. 1990. *Awareness*. New York: Doubleday.

From the publisher: "Using humor, compassion, and insight, the beloved and best-selling Anthony de Mello teaches us to welcome the challenge of knowing ourselves and living the 'aware' life. Mixing Christian spirituality, Buddhist parables, Islamic sayings, Hindu breathing exercises, and psychological insight, spiritualist and Jesuit priest Anthony de Mello challenges readers to identify our most submerged, darkest feelings, accept them, not let them rule us, and allow this new awareness of ourselves to change us."

Kabat-Zinn, J. 1995. *Wherever You Go, There You Are*. New York: Hyperion Books.

A primer on the principles of mindfulness that blends stories, poems, images, and scientific observations with instructions in the art of "capturing" the present and living fully within each moment to achieve inner peace.

Nhat Hahn, T. 1999. *The Miracle of Mindfulness*. Boston, Mass.: Beacon Press.

From the publisher: "Zen master Nhat Hanh weaves practical instruction with anecdotes and other stories to show how the meditative mind can be achieved at all times and how it can help us all 'reveal and heal.' Nhat Hanh is a master at helping us find a calm refuge within ourselves and teaching us how to reach out from there to the rest of the world."

Personal Accounts

Reiland, R. 2004. *Get Me Out of Here! My Recovery from Borderline Personality Disorder.* Center City, Minn.: Hazelden.
From the publisher: "Borderline Personality Disorder. 'What the hell was that?' raged Rachel Reiland when she read the diagnosis written in her medical chart. As the 29-year-old accountant, wife, and mother of young children would soon discover, it was the diagnosis that finally explained her explosive anger, manipulative behaviors, and self-destructive episodes."

Van Gelder, K. 2010. *The Buddha and the Borderline: My Recovery from Borderline Personality Disorder through Dialectical Behavior Therapy, Buddhism, and Online Dating.* Oakland, Calif.: New Harbinger Publications.
From the publisher: "*The Buddha and the Borderline* is a window into this mysterious and debilitating condition, an unblinking portrayal of one woman's fight against the emotional devastation of borderline personality disorder. This haunting, intimate memoir chronicles both the devastating period that led to Kiera's eventual diagnosis and her inspirational recovery through therapy, Buddhist spirituality, and a few online dates gone wrong. Kiera's story sheds light on the private struggle to transform suffering into compassion for herself and others, and is essential reading for all seeking to understand what it truly means to recover and reclaim the desire to live."

Johnson, M. L. 2010. *Girl in Need of a Tourniquet: Memoir of a Borderline Personality.* Berkeley, Calif.: Seal Press.
From the publisher: "An honest and compelling memoir . . . Johnson describes the feeling of 'bleeding out'—unable to tell where she stopped and where her partner began. A self-confessed 'psycho girlfriend,' she was influenced by many emotional factors from her past. She recalls her path through a dysfunctional, destructive relationship, while recounting the experiences that brought her to her breaking point. In recognizing her struggle with borderline personality disorder, Johnson is ultimately able to seek help, embarking on a soul-searching healing process. It's a path that is painful, difficult, and at times heart-wrenching, but ultimately makes her more able to love and coexist in healthy relationships."

Therapy Manuals

Linehan, M. M. 1993. *Skills Training Manual for Treating Borderline Personality Disorder.* New York: Guilford Press.
A step-by step guide for teaching four sets of skills: mindfulness, interpersonal effectiveness, emotion regulation, and distress tolerance. It includes useful, clear-cut handouts that can be readily photocopied.

Bateman, A., and P. Fonagy. 2006. *Mentalization-Based Treatment for Borderline Personality Disorder: A Practical Guide.* Oxford: Oxford University Press.

Miller, A. L., J. H. Rathus, and M. Linehan. 2007. *Dialectical Behavior Therapy with Suicidal Adolescents.* New York: Guilford Press.

Yeomans, F. E., J. F. Clarkin, and O. F. Kernberg. 2002. *A Primer on Transference-Focused Psychotherapy for the Borderline Patient.* Northvale, N.J.: J. Aronson.

The Perspectives of Psychiatry

McHugh, P. R., and P. R. Slavney. 1998. *The Perspectives of Psychiatry,* 2nd ed. Baltimore: Johns Hopkins University Press.
From the publisher: "Paul R. McHugh and Phillip R. Slavney offer an approach that emphasizes psychiatry's unifying concepts while accommodating its diversity. Recognizing that there may never be a single, all-encompassing theory, the book distills psychiatric practice into four explanatory methods: diseases, dimensions of personality, goal-directed behaviors, and life stories. These perspectives, argue the authors, underlie the principles and practice of all psychiatry. With an understanding of these fundamental methods, readers will be equipped to organize and evaluate psychiatric information and to develop a confident approach to practice and research."

APPENDIX B

Theory and Development of the Borderline Concept

A Primer for Students and Therapists

In 1921, Emil Kraepelin's *Manic-Depressive Insanity* was first published in English translation, extracted from his much larger *Textbook of Psychiatry*, the first edition of which had appeared in Germany in the previous century. In this text, he published descriptions of personality characteristics that tend to occur in patients afflicted with manic-depressive syndrome. One of these was the "excitable" or "irritable" personality:

> The patients display from youth up extraordinarily great fluctuations in emotional equilibrium and are greatly moved by all experiences, frequently in an unpleasant way . . . They flare up, and on the most trivial occasion fall into outbursts of boundless fury. The coloring of mood is subject to frequent change . . . periods are interpolated in which they are irritable and ill-humored, also perhaps sad, spiritless, anxious; they shed tears without cause, give expression to thoughts of suicide, bring forward hypochondriacal complaints . . . They are mostly very distractible and unsteady in their endeavors. In consequence of their irritability and their changing moods their conduct of life is subject to the most multifarious incidents, they make sudden resolves, and carry them out on the spot, run off abruptly, go traveling, enter a cloister.[1]

In this description, Kraepelin describes many features commonly encountered in persons who have borderline personality disorder, including impulsivity, unstable relationships, inappropriate and intense anger, affective instability, and physically self-damaging acts.[2]

Kraepelin, who was professor of psychiatry at the University of Heidelberg and later the University of Munich, produced hugely influential works on mental illness at the end of the nineteenth century, works that continue to form the basis for modern classification systems in psychiatry. Although he used the term "personality" in talking about these patients, he saw their problems as an extension of the same "morbid process" that caused the symptoms of manic-depressive illness.

> We include here [in manic-depressive insanity] certain slight and slightest colorings of mood, some of them periodic, some of them continuously morbid, which on the one hand are to be regarded as the rudiment of more severe disorders; on the other hand, *pass without sharp boundary into the domain of personal predisposition.* (emphasis added)

The rise of Freudian psychoanalytic theory, which started to dominate the theoretical orientation of English and American psychiatrists starting in the 1920s, diminished the influence of earlier German theorists and their emphasis on biological factors as the primary etiological factors in psychiatric disease, an influence that met its demise in the ashes of World War II. By the middle of the twentieth century, psychoanalytic thinking completely dominated psychiatry and clinical psychology. Unsurprisingly, when mid-twentieth-century psychiatrists took up the effort to understand these challenging patients, they based their theoretical concepts entirely in terms of psychoanalytic theory.

Freudian followers speak of personality "organization," and propose that all individuals function at one of three levels of personality organization: normal, neurotic, or psychotic. Psychotic organization is the most rudimentary, in which even the most basic ego defense mechanism, reality testing (the ability to distinguish what occurs in one's own mind from what is occurring in the external world), often breaks down. Neurotic organization is a higher, more mature level; patients with neurotic illnesses (characterized mostly by anxiety) are more functional, and it is proposed that they have more mature forms of ego defense.

Freud created these classifications as a way to explain the efficacy of psychoanalysis in some patients and its failure in others, proposing that patients with schizophrenia and other psychoses were untreatable by traditional psychoanalysis because of the level of ego dysfunction present in patients with psychotic personality organization. Patients with at least a neurotic level of organization, on the other hand, could benefit because of their more intact ego functioning and their ability to form a transference relationship in analysis.

As time progressed, psychoanalysts began to recognize a group of patients who had many characteristics of persons with neuroses, but who were highly resistant to psychoanalytic treatment. Some psychoanalysts proposed that these patients, despite their apparent level of ego functioning at a neurotic level, had a mild form of schizophrenia, and coined terms such as *latent schizophrenia* and *pseudo-neurotic schizophrenia* to characterize them.

In 1938, the psychologist Adolf Stern wrote a paper entitled "Psychoanalytic Investigation of and Therapy in the Borderline Group of Neuroses,"[3] proposing instead that these patients were lower-functioning neurotics. He described them as characterized by quickness to anger, depression, and anxiety in response to analytic attempts to make interpretations about their self-esteem; the predominant use of projection as an ego defense (attributing their own internal anger to hostile sources in the environment); extreme narcissism; and difficulties in (but not a failure of) reality testing.

The term *borderline* came to be used among analysts to describe a subset of patients who seemed superficially to have a neurotic personality organization but were less able to function and, most important, highly resistant to traditional analytic techniques. In 1942, Helene Deutsch described individuals whose psychological functioning was characterized by emotional passivity and emptiness and who were capable of only superficial relationships. She had previously coined the term "As if" personality to capture the lack of a secure sense of self in these patients.

Other early descriptions of these persons noted that they "lead a chaotic life in which something dreadful is always happening" (Schmideberg 1947), developed "parasitic" relationships (Rado 1956), and showed "chaotic sexuality, often with frigidity and promiscuity combined" (Esser and Lesser 1965).[4]

In 1967, Otto Kernberg, one of the few psychoanalysts who did not consider these patients essentially untreatable, dove headfirst into the difficulties posed by their treatment. He proposed that these individuals suffered from what could be understood as arising from a failure of their ego structure to fully develop, leading them to compensate by behaving in self-destructive ways. He felt that the only appropriate way in which to understand them was to consider them an entirely new category of personality organization, one whose "underlying psychology does not have the chaos, disorganization, or defect in reality testing associated with psychotic patients, but also lacks the integration, stability of relationships, and regulation of affect associated with neurotic patients."[5]

Borderline patients, he argued, were identified most clearly by their identity diffusion (rather than impaired reality testing) and the use of primitive defense mechanisms. These patients "present contradictory characteristics, chaotic co-existence of defenses against and direct expression of primitive 'id contents' in consciousness, a kind of pseudo-insight into their personality without real concern for nor awareness of the conflictual nature of the material, and a lack of clear identity and lack of understanding in depth of other people." He proposed that these patients cannot develop a stable transference with a therapist because they have little fixed (or integrated) sense of self on which to anchor those representations. The major implication of his formulation was that patients with borderline personality organization could in fact be treated with psychoanalytic psychotherapy, though only with a highly modified version. This approach would later form the backbone of his transference-focused psychotherapy.

In 1972, the psychiatrist James Masterson published a book that contained an extended case study of a single adolescent patient treated by a psychiatric resident on an inpatient unit he had supervised over a period of several years.[6] Masterson noted recurring themes of fear of abandonment and an insatiable desire for nurturing during the patient's treatment and proposed that it was these unmet emotional needs that had stunted her emotional growth. He attempted to focus therapy on successfully negotiating the patient's emotional separation from parents but noted that there was resistance to this process, not only from the patient but also from her parents! He concluded that all of them would need to be "patients" if the therapy was to be successful.

Masterson proposed that a fundamental difficulty in the family system of these patients was "abandonment depression," which prevented the adolescent from severing her emotional dependence on her parents and from developing an independent identity, a developmental process that previous psychoanalytic writers had termed *separation-individuation*. To avoid the deep pain inherent in this process, both patient and parents formed a complicated web of deception and emotional dysfunction that he called *symbiotic*.

Masterson therefore refocused treatment on the parent-child relationship and the emotional pain of separation, which he rather luridly called an "abscess" in the family and noted that the therapist must be wary as the defenses of both the family and the patient "become more frantic" when the separation issues are approached. "When [the therapist] does reach the 'abscess', and lays bare the symbiosis and depression, the family re-experiences their original pain and suffering." Though a particularly intense therapeutic process, he notes that the resulting "catharsis . . . drainage of the 'abscess' relieves the anxiety and depression," and that from that point on, therapy can focus on creating a new, more positive relationship within the family. He found the therapy of this particular patient to be successful, and then expanded it to the entire inpatient unit in the hospital where he worked.

His nearly three-hundred-page book on the subject details other specific patient examples, which are used to illustrate particular therapeutic techniques and successes.

By focusing on the development behind the borderline personality organization, Masterson continued in Kernberg's view of borderline personality disorder as a complex but understandable and fixable condition. Unlike Kernberg, he expanded the scope of treatment in adolescents to include family members and to focus on incomplete parental separation in adults.

In the 1960s, borderline personality disorder became an increasingly common term in psychiatry, no longer confined to obscure psychoanalytic writings but well on its way to recognition as a disorder by American psychiatrists. Unfortunately, however, the therapeutic optimism of Kernberg and Masterson was often ignored, and instead the focus was on the difficulties of treating these patients with psychotherapy. For therapists unable or unwilling to muster the "patient, tolerant, vigilant and persistent" stance that Masterson felt was a necessary requirement for the "wearying and traumatic" process of treating them, these patients remained untreatable. Soon, it was common to hear any difficult or unpleasant patient referred to as "borderline," and the term became increasingly pejorative in its connotations. The label not only incorrectly attributed a severe personality disorder to many patients with other problems but was used to excuse therapeutic nihilism in any challenging patient.

This untherapeutic and also highly unscientific set of beliefs and attitudes about these patients was evident to at least one psychoanalyst at the time, who set out to change them. Dr. Roy R. Grinker, who incidentally was one of the last persons to have been psychoanalyzed by Freud himself, published a 1968 study of hospitalized patients who "displayed symptoms consistent with classic borderline descriptions," including poor interpersonal functioning outside the hospital and prior treatment failures, but who had intact reality testing. Rather than attempting to explain the reasons for their symptoms and behaviors by analyzing them, Grinker and his associates simply observed and recorded them, eventually identifying nearly one hundred symptoms and behavioral variables in these patients and using factor analysis to define subcategories of borderline personality presentations.[7]

Grinker and colleagues proposed that anger and depression were the most salient emotions for these patients. Their anger "expressed more or less directly to a variety of targets . . . seems to constitute the main or only affect that the borderline patient experiences." They proposed that the expression of this anger and the patient's maladaptive psychological defenses against it were major discriminating features of these patients. The other predominant affect of these patients, depression, they described as "not the typical guilt-laden, self-accusatory, remorseful 'end-of-the-rope' type, but more a loneliness as the subjects realize their predicament of being unable to commit themselves in a world of transacting individuals."

In 1975, Drs. John Gunderson and Margaret Singer published a comprehensive review of previously published descriptions of patients who had borderline personality organization, and proposed that six features of their affective experiences and individual and interpersonal behaviors could be used to define the disorder: (1) the presence of intense affect, usually of a strongly hostile or depressed nature; (2) impulsive behaviors, including both episodic acts like self-mutilation and repeated suicide attempts, as well as ongoing patterns such as addiction or sexual promiscuity; (3) superficial social adaptation manifested by achievement in school or work, appropriate appearance and manners, and strong social awareness that nevertheless masked a disturbed identity; (4) brief psychotic experiences usually of a paranoid quality that usually arose during drug use or in the setting of unstructured situations and relationships; (5) characteristic findings on psychological testing, with patients giving bizarre, illogical, or primitive responses on unstructured tests such as the Rorschach, but not on more structured tests such as the WAIS; and (6) dysfunctional interpersonal relationships that typically vacillated between transient, superficial relationships and intense, dependent relationships marred by manipulation.[8]

Based on these characteristics, Gunderson and his colleagues developed a research interview tool that they proposed could identify the syndrome of borderline personality and differentiate it from other personality organizations with "a high degree of accuracy."[9]

In no small degree as a result of Gunderson's work, enough of a consensus within the psychiatric community developed to adopt specific criteria for defining borderline personality disorder, the category appearing in the third edition of the American Psychiatric Association's *Diagnostic and Statistical Manual of Mental Disorders* in 1980.

But although borderline personality disorder now had clearly defined diagnostic criteria, the concept remained intuitively unsatisfying from a more scientific perspective for many. There was nothing in any of the DSM's diagnostic criteria that reflected the previous fifty years of work by the likes of Kernberg and Masterson in understanding and defining it, albeit in terms of personality organization and ego functioning rather than observable symptoms and behaviors. In 1985, a leading researcher on mood disorders published an article titled, "Borderline: An Adjective in Search of a Noun," and reported that when his team had evaluated one hundred outpatients with the borderline diagnosis, they had met DSM diagnostic criteria for a whole panoply of other diagnostic categories; he argued that the term borderline "does not identify a specific psychopathologic syndrome." Training at Johns Hopkins in the early 1980s, one of us usually heard the diagnosis referred to as the "so-called borderline personality disorder."

Despite this uncertainty and disagreement within the field, however, researchers continued to study these patients and increasingly to use methods other than psychoanalysis to understand them. Family and genetic studies, neuroimaging work, and other biologically informed studies began to appear.

In 1991, Siever and Davis published "A Psychobiological Perspective on the Personality Disorders," in which they proposed two underlying biological mechanisms for these conditions.[10] First, they suggested that overactivity of noradrenergic circuits in the brain caused these patients to have chronic *affective instability*, making them prone "to marked, rapidly reversible shifts in affective state that are extremely sensitive to meaningful environmental events that might induce more modest emotional responses in other people." Since "representations of self and others may be influenced by affective state, an instability in mood may impair an individual's capacity to maintain a stable self-esteem. Such individuals may develop coping and defense mechanisms to minimize the impact of their affective sensitivity . . . [they] may exaggerate their affective responses, using their emotionality to control the behavior of others in order to modulate their own mood and self-esteem. Such individuals often do not perceive their behavior as manipulative but as essential to the maintenance of their affective well-being." They proposed that the decreased REM onset latency during sleep and "hyper-responsiveness to catecholeminergic drugs," such as amphetamines, that had been observed in patients diagnosed with borderline personality were biological correlates of this underlying hyperadrenergic neural state.

Second, Siever and Davis suggested that reduced serotonergic modulation in these patients put them at high risk for *behavioral dyscontrol*, a decreased ability to tolerate external or internal stimuli without acting, resulting in problems such as impulsivity and aggression. They "have difficulty anticipating the effects of their behavior . . . tend to externalize the source of their difficulties, are prone to excessive expression of aggression and frustration . . . In borderline personality disorders, impulsivity/aggression may be expressed as suicide attempts, angry outbursts, fights, and substance abuse, often in response to a disappointment or frustration in an important relationship." Animal models had demonstrated increases in violent behavior as a result of experimental lesions in serotonergic centers, and reduced amounts of serotonin byproducts had been found in the cerebrospinal fluid of patients who had attempted suicide, patients with a history of violent and aggressive behaviors, and "in violent offenders." Proposed biological correlates of serotonergic dysfunction that had already been observed in borderline patients included excess EEG slow-wave activity in the brain and a reduced pituitary prolactin response to the serotonergic-releasing agent fenfluramine.

An additional appeal of these proposals was that they offered a way to explain the observed similarities of the symptoms and behaviors of these patients to those of persons with illness of more clearly biological etiology, especially bipolar disorder. Dr. Dean MacKinnon of Johns Hopkins published an elegant explanatory model of the continuity between borderline personality disorder and bipolar disorder based on the similar biological findings in both sets of patients as well as on the fact that anticonvulsant mood-stabilizer medications have shown promise in the treatment of these patients (figure B.1).

The vulnerability to both unstable mood states (e.g., rapid-cycling bipolar disorder) and to unstable temperaments may derive from genetics or other insult to the optimal emotional functioning of the brain. In figure B.1, shaded arrows illustrate the vicious cycle by which the combination of temperamental vulnerability and unsupportive environment can lead to frank affective symptomatology. Pathological or inappropriate affective states affect the child's reward/punishment perception directly, and in a reciprocal way, by leading to a cycle of conduct problems and inconsistent parenting and persistently conflicted parental relationship, which in turn adversely influences psychological development. All these factors produce stress, which adversely affects brain systems involved in mood regulation through corticosteroidal mechanisms. The cumulative effect of this cycle is more mood dysregulation and worsening problems with the affective and behavioral symptoms, as well as the problems with relationships and psychological integrity typical of borderline personality disorder.

Open arrows in figure B.1 illustrate a typical, relatively uncomplicated case of familial bipolar disorder. The patient experiences a cycle from temperamental vulnerability to life problems, influenced by impairment in reward perception, leading to stressful situations, with the resulting harmful effects of stress on brain functions involved with maintenance of affective stability. If severe parent-child difficulties do not occur, however (the blocked arrow), the second loop of the cycle is avoided, and the person does not develop a personality disorder. Factors that would block this second cycle might include high parental resiliency and resourcefulness; protective temperamental features in the child (e.g., conscientiousness, stoicism),

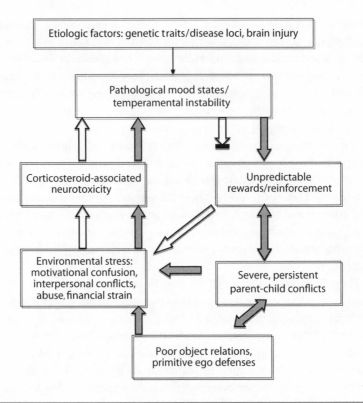

Figure B.I. A Bio-developmental model for borderline personality disorder and the bipolar spectrum. Modified from D. F. MacKinnon and R. Pies, "Affective instability as rapid cycling: Theoretical and clinical implications for borderline personality and bipolar spectrum disorders," *Bipolar Disorders* 8 (2006): 1–14.

or prolonged periods of relative affective calm when healthy psychological development can proceed.

Similar ideas inform most theories on the etiology of borderline personality disorder now and represent a truly bio-psycho-social understanding of this complex disorder.

In addition to the development of new theoretical approaches to the disorder, many more data have been gathered on epidemiology and illness course.

Enormous amounts of new data on the phenomenology, epidemiology, and natural history of BPD are now available thanks to two landmark longitudinal studies, the Collaborative Longitudinal Study of Personality Disorders[11] and the McLean Study of Adult Development.[12] As a result of these studies, it is now clearer and more widely accepted that the natural history of the disorder is usually quite favorable, with a substantial proportion of persons who have BPD recovering from the most disabling features of the disorder, albeit over a period of years.

In April 2008, the U.S. House of Representatives unanimously passed House Resolution 1005 supporting the month of May as borderline personality disorder awareness month. The resolution stated that "despite its prevalence, enormous public health costs, and the devastating toll it takes on individuals, families, and communities, [borderline personality disorder] only recently has begun to command the attention it requires."[13]

Last, in addition to controlled clinical trials of pharmacological approaches, empirical testing of several manualized therapies has now started, again with promising results. All these therapies draw on successful time-tested models, psychodynamic psychotherapy and cognitive behavioral therapy (CBT). Unfortunately, only one among them, dialectical behavioral therapy (DBT), has developed anything approaching easy availability for most patients.

Nevertheless, both etiological and therapeutic research continues furiously and internationally, making it possible to be quite optimistic about the development of increasingly effective treatments for these patients. The future appears bright for them and for those caring for them.

REFERENCES

INTRODUCTION

1. Zanarini, M. C., F. R. Frankenburg, J. Hennen, D. B. Reich, and K. R. Silk. 2005. "The McLean study of adult development (MSAD): Overview and implications of the first six years of prospective follow-up." *Journal of Personality Disorders* 19 (5) (Oct.): 505–23.
2. Cloud, J. 2009. "The Mystery of Borderline Personality Disorder." *Time.* January 8.
3. Morton, A. 1998. *Diana: Her True Story in Her Own Words.* Revised ed. New York: Simon and Schuster; Pocket.
4. Packer-Fletcher, D. 2000. "Diana in search of herself: Portrait of a troubled princess." *Psychiatric Services* 51 (2) (February 1): 259–60.

CHAPTER 1. THE CLINICAL PICTURE

1. Anonymous. My journey with BPD [cited 10/21/2008]. Available from www .mhsanctuary.com/borderline/journey.htm (accessed 10/21/2008).
2. Reiland, R. 2004. *Get Me Out of Here: My Recovery from Borderline Personality Disorder.* Center City, MN: Hazelden.
3. Anonymous. My personal borderline personality disorder story. Available from www.angelfire.com/biz/BPD/story.html (accessed 10/21/2008).
4. Park, K. Greetings from the bottom. Available from www.mhsanctuary .com/borderline/greetings.htm (accessed 10/21/2008).
5. National Collaborating Centre for Mental Health. 2009. *Borderline Personality Disorder: Treatment and Management.* London: British Psychological Society and the Royal College of Psychiatrists, 69.
6. Shedler, J., and D. Westen. 2007. "The Shedler-Westen assessment procedure (SWAP): Making personality diagnosis clinically meaningful." *Journal of Personality Assessment* 89 (1) (Aug.): 41–55.
7. Zittel Conklin, C., and D. Westen. 2005. "Borderline personality disorder in clinical practice." *American Journal of Psychiatry* 162 (5) (May): 867–75.

CHAPTER 2. "PERSONALITY" AND MORE

1. Ryckman, R. M. 2008. *Theories of Personality*. 9th ed. Florence, KY: Cengage Learning, 4.
2. Jaspers, K. 1997. *General Psychopathology*. Baltimore: Johns Hopkins University Press, 428.
3. Thomas, A. R., and S. Chess. 1968. *Temperament and Behavior Disorders in Children*. New York: New York University Press, 23.
4. Pedlow, R., A. Sanson, M. Prior, and F. Oberklaid. 1993. "Stability of maternally reported temperament from infancy to 8 years." *Developmental Psychology* 29 (6) (11): 998–1007.
5. Alliance of Psychoanalytic Organizations. 2006. *Psychodynamic Diagnostic Manual*. Silver Spring, MD: Interdisciplinary Council on Developmental and Learning Disorders, 18.
6. Gunderson, J. G., R. L. Stout, C. A. Sanislow, M. T. Shea, T. H. McGlashan, M. C. Zanarini, M. T. Daversa, C. M. Grilo, S. Yen, and A. E. Skodol. 2008. "New episodes and new onsets of major depression in borderline and other personality disorders." *Journal of Affective Disorders* 111 (1) (11): 40–45.
7. Zanarini, M. C., F. R. Frankenburg, D. B. Reich, G. Fitzmaurice, I. Weinberg, and J. G. Gunderson. 2008. "The 10-year course of physically self-destructive acts reported by borderline patients and axis II comparison subjects." *Acta Psychiatrica Scandinavica* 117 (3) (Mar): 177–84.
8. Grant, B. F., S. P. Chou, R. B. Goldstein, B. Huang, F. S. Stinson, T. D. Saha, S. M. Smith, et al. 2008. "Prevalence, correlates, disability, and comorbidity of DSM-IV borderline personality disorder: Results from the wave 2 national epidemiologic survey on alcohol and related conditions." *Journal of Clinical Psychiatry* 69 (4) (April): 533–45.
9. Zanarini, M. C., F. R. Frankenburg, J. Hennen, D. B. Reich, and K. R. Silk. 2004. "Axis I comorbidity in patients with borderline personality disorder: 6-year follow-up and prediction of time to remission." *American Journal of Psychiatry* 161 (11) (Nov.): 2108–14.

CHAPTER 3. THE FOUR FACES OF BORDERLINE PERSONALITY DISORDER

1. Hartwell, C. E. 1996. "The schizophrenogenic mother concept in American psychiatry." *Psychiatry* 59 (3) (Fall): 274–97.
2. McHugh, P. R., and P. R. Slavney. 1998. *The Perspectives of Psychiatry*. Baltimore: Johns Hopkins University Press.

3. Jaspers, K. 1997. *General Psychopathology*. Baltimore: Johns Hopkins University Press, 428.
4. Milne, D. 2003. "Japan grapples with alcoholism crisis." *Psychiatric News* 38 (23) (Dec. 5): 12–57.
5. Jalava, J. 2006. "The modern degenerate: Nineteenth-century degeneration theory and modern psychopathy research." *Theory and Psychology* 16:416–32.

CHAPTER 4. WHAT THE PERSON HAS

1. Styron, W. 1990. *Darkness Visible: A Memoir of Madness*. New York: Random House.
2. Gunderson, J. G., R. L. Stout, C. A. Sanislow, M. T. Shea, T. H. McGlashan, M. C. Zanarini, M. T. Daversa, C. M. Grilo, S. Yen, and A. E. Skodol. 2008. "New episodes and new onsets of major depression in borderline and other personality disorders." *Journal of Affective Disorders* 111 (1) (11): 40–45.
3. Akiskal, H. S., and O. Pinto. 1999. "The evolving bipolar spectrum. Prototypes I, II, III, and IV." *Psychiatric Clinics of North America* 22 (3) (Sept.): 517–34, vii.
4. Gunderson, J. G., I. Weinberg, M. T. Daversa, K. D. Kueppenbender, M. C. Zanarini, M. T. Shea, A. E. Skodol, et al. 2006. "Descriptive and longitudinal observations on the relationship of borderline personality disorder and bipolar disorder." *American Journal of Psychiatry* 163 (7) (July 1): 1173–78.
5. Merikangas, K. R., H. S. Akiskal, J. Angst, P. E. Greenberg, R. M. A. Hirschfeld, M. Petukhova, and R. C. Kessler. 2007. "Lifetime and 12-month prevalence of bipolar spectrum disorder in the national comorbidity survey replication." *Archives of General Psychiatry* 64 (5) (May 1): 543–52.
6. Tritt, K., C. Nickel, C. Lahmann, P. K. Leiberich, W. K. Rother, T. H. Loew, and M. K. Nickel. 2005. "Lamotrigine treatment of aggression in female borderline patients: A randomized, double-blind, placebo-controlled study." *Journal of Psychopharmacology* (Oxford, England) 19 (3) (May): 287–91.
7. Dell'Osso, B., H. A. Berlin, M. Serati, and A. C. Altamura. 2010. "Neuropsychobiological aspects, comorbidity patterns and dimensional models in borderline personality disorder." *Neuropsychobiology* 61 (4): 169–79.
8. Tebartz van Elst, L., P. Ludaescher, T. Thiel, M. Buchert, B. Hesslinger, M. Bohus, N. Rusch, J. Hennig, D. Ebert, and K. Lieb. 2007. "Evidence

of disturbed amygdalar energy metabolism in patients with borderline personality disorder." *Neuroscience Letters* 417 (1) (April 24): 36–41.

9. Donegan, N. H., C. A. Sanislow, H. P. Blumberg, R. K. Fulbright, C. Lacadie, P. Skudlarski, J. C. Gore, I. R. Olson, T. H. McGlashan, and B. E. Wexler. 2003. "Amygdala hyperreactivity in borderline personality disorder: Implications for emotional dysregulation." *Biological Psychiatry* 54 (11) (12/1): 1284–93.

10. Silbersweig, D., J. F. Clarkin, M. Goldstein, O. F. Kernberg, O. Tuescher, K. N. Levy, G. Brendel, et al. 2007. "Failure of frontolimbic inhibitory function in the context of negative emotion in borderline personality disorder." *American Journal of Psychiatry* 164 (12) (Dec.): 1832–41.

11. Kendler, K. S., S. H. Aggen, N. Czajkowski, E. Roysamb, K. Tambs, S. Torgersen, M. C. Neale, and T. Reichborn-Kjennerud. 2008. "The structure of genetic and environmental risk factors for DSM-IV personality disorders: A multivariate twin study." *Archives of General Psychiatry* 65 (12) (Dec.): 1438–46.

12. Zetzsche, T., U. W. Preuss, B. Bondy, T. Frodl, P. Zill, G. Schmitt, N. Koutsouleris, et al. 2008. "5-HT1A receptor gene C-1019 G polymorphism and amygdala volume in borderline personality disorder." *Genes, Brain, and Behavior* 7 (3) (April): 306–13.

CHAPTER 5. THE DIMENSIONS OF BORDERLINE
PERSONALITY DISORDER

1. Allport, G. W., and H. S. Odbert. 1936. "Trait names: A psycholexical study." *Psychology Monographs* 47:211.

2. Cattell, R. B., M. B. Marshall, and S. Georgiades. 1957. "Personality and motivation: Structure and measurement." *Journal of Personality Disorders* 19 (1): 53–67.

3. Tupes, E. C., and R. E. Christal. 1961. *Recurrent Personality Factors Based on Trait Ratings*. Lackland Air Force Base, TX: U.S. Air Force, 61–97.

4. Foulkrod, K. H., C. Field, and C. V. Brown. 2010. "Trauma surgeon personality and job satisfaction: Results from a national survey." *American Surgeon* 76 (4) (April): 422–27.

5. de Bruijn, G. J., J. Brug, and F. J. Van Lenthe. 2009. "Neuroticism, conscientiousness and fruit consumption: Exploring mediator and moderator effects in the theory of planned behaviour." *Psychology & Health* 24 (9) (Nov.): 1051–69.

6. Terracciano, A., and P. T. Costa, Jr. 2004. "Smoking and the five-factor

model of personality." *Addiction* (Abingdon, England) 99 (4) (April): 472–81.

7. Tang, T. Z., R. J. DeRubeis, S. D. Hollon, J. Amsterdam, R. Shelton, and B. Schalet. 2009. "Personality change during depression treatment: A placebo-controlled trial." *Archives of General Psychiatry* 66 (12) (Dec. 1): 1322–30.

8. Hopwood, C. J., M. B. Donnellan, and M. C. Zanarini. 2009. "Temperamental and acute symptoms of borderline personality disorder: Associations with normal personality traits and dynamic relations over time." *Psychological Medicine* (Dec. 17): 1–8.

9. McCrae, R. R., and O. P. John. 1992. "An introduction to the five-factor model and its applications." *Journal of Personality* 60 (2) (June): 175–215.

10. Watson, D., and L. A. Clark. 1984. "Negative affectivity: The disposition to experience aversive emotional states." *Psychological Bulletin* 96 (3) (Nov.): 465–90.

11. Loehlin, J. C., R. R. McCrae, P. T. Costa, and O. P. John. 1998. "Heritabilities of common and measure-specific components of the big five personality factors." *Journal of Research in Personality* 32 (4) (12): 431–53.

12. Roberts, B. W., K. E. Walton, and W. Viechtbauer. 2006. "Patterns of mean-level change in personality traits across the life course: A meta-analysis of longitudinal studies." *Psychological Bulletin* 132 (1) (Jan.): 1–25.

13. Vinnars, B., B. Thormahlen, R. Gallop, K. Noren, and J. P. Barber. 2009. "Do personality problems improve during psychodynamic supportive-expressive psychotherapy? Secondary outcome results from a randomized controlled trial for psychiatric outpatients with personality disorders." *Psychotherapy* (Chicago) 46 (3) (Sept. 1): 362–75.

CHAPTER 6. BEHAVIORS I

1. Brembs, B. 2003. "Operant conditioning in invertebrates." *Current Opinion in Neurobiology* 13 (6) (Dec.): 710–17.

2. McGlashan, T. H., C. M. Grilo, A. E. Skodol, J. G. Gunderson, M. T. Shea, L. C. Morey, M. C. Zanarini, and R. L. Stout. 2000. "The collaborative longitudinal personality disorders study: Baseline axis I/II and II/II diagnostic co-occurrence." *Acta Psychiatrica Scandinavica* 102 (4) (Oct.): 256–64.

3. Walter, M., J. G. Gunderson, M. C. Zanarini, C. A. Sanislow, C. M. Grilo, T. H. McGlashan, L. C. Morey, S. Yen, R. L. Stout, and A. E. Skodol. 2009. "New onsets of substance use disorders in borderline person-

ality disorder over 7 years of follow-ups: Findings from the collaborative longitudinal personality disorders study." *Addiction* 104 (1): 97–103.

4. Johns, A. 2001. "Psychiatric effects of cannabis." *British Journal of Psychiatry* 178 (Feb.): 116–22.

5. Christophersen, A. S. 2000. "Amphetamine designer drugs—an overview and epidemiology." *Toxicology Letters* 112–13 (March 15): 127–31.

6. Sansone, R. A., and M. W. Wiederman. 2009. "The abuse of prescription medications: Borderline personality patients in psychiatric versus non-psychiatric settings." *International Journal of Psychiatry in Medicine* 39 (2): 147–54.

7. Riegel, A. C., and P. W. Kalivas. 2010. "Neuroscience: Lack of inhibition leads to abuse." *Nature* 463 (7282) (Feb. 11): 743–44.

8. Brumberg, J. J. 2000; 1989. *Fasting Girls: The History of Anorexia Nervosa.* 1st Vintage Books ed. New York: Vintage Books.

9. Lasker, G. W. 1947. "The effects of partial starvation on somatotype: An analysis of material from the Minnesota starvation experiment." *American Journal of Physical Anthropology* 5 (3): 323–42.

10. Kreipe, R. E., and S. A. Birndorf. 2000. "Eating disorders in adolescents and young adults." *Medical Clinics of North America* 84 (4) (July): 1027–49, viii–ix.

11. Zanarini, M. C., C. A. Reichman, F. R. Frankenburg, D. B. Reich, and G. Fitzmaurice. 2009. "The course of eating disorders in patients with borderline personality disorder: A 10-year follow-up study." *International Journal of Eating Disorders* 43 (3) (April): 226–32.

12. MacLaren, V. V., and L. A. Best. 2009. "Female students' disordered eating and the big five personality facets." *Eating Behaviors* 10 (3) (8): 192–95.

13. Kong, S., and K. Bernstein. 2009. "Childhood trauma as a predictor of eating psychopathology and its mediating variables in patients with eating disorders." *Journal of Clinical Nursing* 18 (13): 1897–1907.

14. Kröger, C., U. Schweiger, V. Sipos, S. Kliem, R. Arnold, T. Schunert, and H. Reinecker. 2010. "Dialectical behaviour therapy and an added cognitive behavioural treatment module for eating disorders in women with borderline personality disorder and anorexia nervosa or bulimia nervosa who failed to respond to previous treatments: An open trial with a 15-month follow-up." *Journal of Behavior Therapy and Experimental Psychiatry* 41 (4) (12): 381–88.

CHAPTER 7. BEHAVIORS II

1. Egan, J. 1997. "The Thin Red Line." *New York Times Magazine*, July 27.
2. National Collaborating Centre for Mental Health. 2009. *Borderline Personality Disorder: Treatment and Management*. London: British Psychological Society and the Royal College of Psychiatrists, 60.
3. Favazza, A. R. 1998. "The coming of age of self-mutilation." *Journal of Nervous and Mental Disease* 186 (5) (May): 259–68.
4. Zanarini, M. C., F. R. Frankenburg, D. B. Reich, G. Fitzmaurice, I. Weinberg, and J. G. Gunderson. 2008. "The 10-year course of physically self-destructive acts reported by borderline patients and axis II comparison subjects." *Acta Psychiatrica Scandinavica* 117 (3) (March): 177–84.
5. Zanarini, M. C., F. R. Frankenburg, M. E. Ridolfi, S. Jager-Hyman, J. Hennen, and J. G. Gunderson. 2006. "Reported childhood onset of self-mutilation among borderline patients." *Journal of Personality Disorders* 20 (1) (Feb.): 9–15.
6. Klonsky, E. D. 2007. "The functions of deliberate self-injury: A review of the evidence." *Clinical Psychology Review* 27 (2) (March): 226–39.
7. Linehan, M. 1993. *Cognitive-Behavioral Therapy of Borderline Personality Disorder*. New York: The Guilford Press, 144.
8. Frances, A. 1987. "Introduction." *Journal of Personality Disorders* 1 (4) (Winter): 316.
9. Black, D. W., N. Blum, B. Pfohl, and N. Hale. 2004. "Suicidal behavior in borderline personality disorder: Prevalence, risk factors, prediction, and prevention." *Journal of Personality Disorders* 18 (3) (June): 226–39.
10. Yen, S., M. T. Shea, C. A. Sanislow, C. M. Grilo, A. E. Skodol, J. G. Gunderson, T. H. McGlashan, M. C. Zanarini, and L. C. Morey. 2004. "Borderline personality disorder criteria associated with prospectively observed suicidal behavior." *American Journal of Psychiatry* 161 (7) (July): 1296–98.
11. Brown, M. Z., K. A. Comtois, and M. M. Linehan. 2002. "Reasons for suicide attempts and nonsuicidal self-injury in women with borderline personality disorder." *Journal of Abnormal Psychology* 111 (1) (Feb.): 198–202.
12. Sansone, R. A. 2004. "Chronic suicidality and borderline personality." *Journal of Personality Disorders* 18 (3) (June): 215–25.
13. Brodsky, B. S., S. A. Groves, M. A. Oquendo, J. J. Mann, and B. Stanley. 2006. "Interpersonal precipitants and suicide attempts in border-

line personality disorder." *Suicide & Life-Threatening Behavior* 36 (3) (June): 313–22.

14. Morgan, C. A., III, G. Hazlett, S. Wang, E. G. Richardson Jr., P. Schnurr, and S. M. Southwick. 2001. "Symptoms of dissociation in humans experiencing acute, uncontrollable stress: A prospective investigation." *American Journal of Psychiatry* 158 (8) (Aug. 1): 1239–47.

15. Korzekwa, M. I., P. F. Dell, P. S. Links, L. Thabane, and P. Fougere. 2009. "Dissociation in borderline personality disorder: A detailed look." *Journal of Trauma & Dissociation: The Official Journal of the International Society for the Study of Dissociation (ISSD)* 10 (3): 346–67.

16. Pope, H. G., Jr., S. Barry, A. Bodkin, and J. I. Hudson. 2006. "Tracking scientific interest in the dissociative disorders: A study of scientific publication output 1984–2003." *Psychotherapy and Psychosomatics* 75 (1): 19–24.

17. Zanarini, M. C. 2000. "Childhood experiences associated with the development of borderline personality disorder." *Psychiatric Clinics of North America* 23 (1) (March): 89–101.

18. Zanarini, M. C., T. F. Ruser, F. R. Frankenburg, J. Hennen, and J. G. Gunderson. 2000. "Risk factors associated with the dissociative experiences of borderline patients." *Journal of Nervous and Mental Disease* 188 (1) (Jan.): 26–30.

CHAPTER 8. THE LIFE STORY

1. Walsh, F. 1977. The family of the borderline patient. In *The Borderline Patient*, eds. R. Grinker, B. Werble, 168–77. New York: Jason Aronson.

2. Zanarini, M. C., A. A. Williams, R. E. Lewis, R. B. Reich, S. C. Vera, M. F. Marino, A. Levin, L. Yong, and F. R. Frankenburg. 1997. "Reported pathological childhood experiences associated with the development of borderline personality disorder." *American Journal of Psychiatry* 154 (8) (Aug. 1): 1101–6.

3. Gunderson, J. G., and A. N. Sabo. 1993. "The phenomenological and conceptual interface between borderline personality disorder and PTSD." *American Journal of Psychiatry* 150 (1) (Jan.): 19–27.

4. Zanarini, M. C., L. Yong, F. R. Frankenburg, J. Hennen, D. B. Reich, M. F. Marino, and A. A. Vujanovic. 2002. "Severity of reported childhood sexual abuse and its relationship to severity of borderline psychopathology and psychosocial impairment among borderline inpatients." *Journal of Nervous and Mental Disease* 190 (6) (June): 381–87.

5. Zanarini, M. C., F. R. Frankenburg, J. Hennen, D. B. Reich, and K. R. Silk. 2004. "Axis I comorbidity in patients with borderline personality dis-

order: 6-year follow-up and prediction of time to remission." *American Journal of Psychiatry* 161 (11) (Nov.): 2108–14.

6. Golier, J. A., R. Yehuda, L. M. Bierer, V. Mitropoulou, A. S. New, J. Schmeidler, J. M. Silverman, and L. J. Siever. 2003. "The relationship of borderline personality disorder to post-traumatic stress disorder and traumatic events." *American Journal of Psychiatry* 160 (11) (Nov. 1): 2018–24.

7. Jovev, M., and H. J. Jackson. 2006. "The relationship of borderline personality disorder, life events and functioning in an Australian psychiatric sample." *Journal of Personality Disorders* 20 (3) (June): 205–17.

CHAPTER 9. TREATING THE DISEASE

1. American Psychiatric Association Practice Guidelines. 2001. "Practice guideline for the treatment of patients with borderline personality disorder: American psychiatric association." *American Journal of Psychiatry* 158 (10 supp.) (Oct.): 1–52.

2. Oldham, J. M. 2005. Guideline watch: Practice guideline for the treatment of patients with borderline personality disorder. In American Psychiatric Association [database online]. Arlington, VA. Available from www.psych.org/psych_pract/treatg/pg/prac_guide.cfm (accessed 9/12/2010).

3. National Collaborating Centre for Mental Health. *Borderline Personality Disorder: Treatment and Management.* London: British Psychological Society and the Royal College of Psychiatrists, 2009, 74, 69.

4. Lieb, K., B. Vollm, G. Rucker, A. Timmer, and J. M. Stoffers. 2010. "Pharmacotherapy for borderline personality disorder: Cochrane systematic review of randomised trials." *British Journal of Psychiatry* 196 (1) (Jan. 1): 4–12.

5. Kendall, T., R. Burbeck, and A. Bateman. 2010. "Pharmacotherapy for borderline personality disorder: NICE guideline." *British Journal of Psychiatry* 196 (2) (Feb. 1): 158–59.

6. Bellino, S., E. Paradiso, and F. Bogetto. 2008. "Efficacy and tolerability of pharmacotherapies for borderline personality disorder." *CNS Drugs* 22 (8): 671–92.

7. Glowinski, J., and J. Axelrod. 1964. "Inhibition of uptake of tritiated-noradrenaline in the intact rat brain by imipramine and structurally related compounds." *Nature* 204 (Dec. 26): 1318–19.

8. Lemberger, L., H. Rowe, R. Carmichael, R. Crabtree, J. S. Horng, F. Bymaster, and D. Wong. 1978. "Fluoxetine, a selective serotonin uptake

inhibitor." *Clinical Pharmacology and Therapeutics* 23 (4) (April): 421–29.

9. Kuhn, R. 1958. "The treatment of depressive states with G 22355 (imipramine hydrochloride)." *American Journal of Psychiatry* 115 (5) (Nov.): 459–64.

10. Soloff, P. H., A. George, S. Nathan, P. M. Schulz, J. R. Cornelius, J. Herring, and J. M. Perel. 1989. "Amitriptyline versus haloperidol in borderlines: Final outcomes and predictors of response." *Journal of Clinical Psychopharmacology* 9 (4) (Aug.): 238–46.

11. Links, P. S., M. Steiner, I. Boiago, and D. Irwin. 1990. "Lithium therapy for borderline patients: Preliminary findings." *Journal of Personality Disorders* 4 (2): 173–81.

12. Soloff, P. H., A. George, R. S. Nathan, P. M. Schulz, R. F. Ulrich, and J. M. Perel. 1986. "Progress in pharmacotherapy of borderline disorders: A double-blind study of amitriptyline, haloperidol, and placebo." *Archives of General Psychiatry* 43 (7) (July): 691–97.

13. Crane, G. E. 1957. "Iproniazid (marsilid) phosphate, a therapeutic agent for mental disorders and debilitating diseases." *Psychiatric Research Reports* 8 (Dec.): 142–52.

14. Parsons, B., F. M. Quitkin, P. J. McGrath, J. W. Stewart, E. Tricamo, K. Ocepek-Welikson, W. Harrison, J. G. Rabkin, S. G. Wager, and E. Nunes. 1989. "Phenelzine, imipramine, and placebo in borderline patients meeting criteria for atypical depression." *Psychopharmacology Bulletin* 25 (4): 524–34.

15. Soloff, P. H., J. Cornelius, A. George, S. Nathan, J. M. Perel, and R. F. Ulrich. 1993. "Efficacy of phenelzine and haloperidol in borderline personality disorder." *Archives of General Psychiatry* 50 (5) (May 1): 377–85.

16. Cornelius, J. R., P. H. Soloff, J. M. Perel, and R. F. Ulrich. 1993. "Continuation pharmacotherapy of borderline personality disorder with haloperidol and phenelzine." *American Journal of Psychiatry* 150 (12) (Dec.): 1843–48.

17. Abraham, P. F., and J. R. Calabrese. 2008. "Evidenced-based pharmacologic treatment of borderline personality disorder: A shift from SSRIs to anticonvulsants and atypical antipsychotics?" *Journal of Affective Disorders* 111 (1) (Nov.): 21–30.

18. Cade, J. F. 1949. "Lithium salts in the treatment of psychotic excitement." *Medical Journal of Australia* 2 (10) (Sept. 3): 349–52.

19. Pinto, O. C., and H. S. Akiskal. 1998. "Lamotrigine as a promising approach to borderline personality: An open case series without concurrent

DSM-IV major mood disorder." *Journal of Affective Disorders* 51 (3) (Dec.): 333–43.

20. Preston, G. A., B. K. Marchant, F. W. Reimherr, R. E. Strong, and D. W. Hedges. 2004. "Borderline personality disorder in patients with bipolar disorder and response to lamotrigine." *Journal of Affective Disorders* 79 (1–3) (April): 297–303.

21. Tritt, K., C. Nickel, C. Lahmann, P. K. Leiberich, W. K. Rother, T. H. Loew, and M. K. Nickel. 2005. "Lamotrigine treatment of aggression in female borderline patients: A randomized, double-blind, placebo-controlled study." *Journal of Psychopharmacology* (Oxford, England) 19 (3) (May): 287–91.

22. Reich, D. B., M. C. Zanarini, and K. A. Bieri. 2009. "A preliminary study of lamotrigine in the treatment of affective instability in borderline personality disorder." *International Clinical Psychopharmacology* 24 (5) (Sept.): 270–75.

23. Faltus, F. J. 1984. "The positive effect of alprazolam in the treatment of three patients with borderline personality disorder." *American Journal of Psychiatry* 141 (6) (June): 802–803.

24. Gardner, D. L., and R. W. Cowdry. 1985. "Alprazolam-induced dyscontrol in borderline personality disorder." *American Journal of Psychiatry* 142 (1) (Jan.): 98–100.

25. Vorma, H., H. H. Naukkarinen, S. J. Sarna, and K. I. Kuoppasalmi. 2005. "Predictors of benzodiazepine discontinuation in subjects manifesting complicated dependence." *Substance Use & Misuse* 40 (4): 499–510.

CHAPTER 10. TREATING THE BEHAVIORS

1. Prochaska, J. O., and W. F. Velicer. 1997. "The transtheoretical model of health behavior change." *American Journal of Health Promotion* 12 (1): 38–48.

2. Beck, A. 1967. *Depression: Causes and Treatment.* Philadelphia: University of Pennsylvania Press.

3. Evans, K., P. Tyrer, J. Catalan, U. Schmidt, K. Davidson, J. Dent, P. Tata, S. Thornton, J. Barber, and S. Thompson. 1999. "Manual-assisted cognitive-behaviour therapy (MACT): A randomized controlled trial of a brief intervention with bibliotherapy in the treatment of recurrent deliberate self-harm." *Psychological Medicine* 29 (1) (Jan.): 19–25.

4. Brown, G. K., C. F. Newman, S. E. Charlesworth, P. Crits-Christoph, and A. T. Beck. 2004. "An open clinical trial of cognitive therapy for borderline personality disorder." *Journal of Personality Disorders* 18 (3) (June): 257–71.

5. Linehan, M. M. 1987. "Dialectical behavior therapy for borderline personality disorder: Theory and method." *Bulletin of the Menninger Clinic* 51 (3) (May): 261–76.

6. Linehan, M. 1993. *Cognitive-Behavioral Therapy of Borderline Personality Disorder.* New York: Guilford Press, 51.

7. Linehan, M. M., H. E. Armstrong, A. Suarez, D. Allmon, and H. L. Heard. 1991. "Cognitive-behavioral treatment of chronically parasuicidal borderline patients." *Archives of General Psychiatry* 48 (12) (Dec. 1): 1060–64.

8. Linehan, M. M. 1995. "Combining pharmacotherapy with psychotherapy for substance abusers with borderline personality disorder: Strategies for enhancing compliance." *NIDA Research Monograph* 150: 129–42.

CHAPTER 11. UNDERSTANDING THE DIMENSIONS AND ADDRESSING THE LIFE STORY

1. Blagys, M. D., and M. J. Hilsenroth. 2000. "Distinctive features of short-term psychodynamic-interpersonal psychotherapy: A review of the comparative psychotherapy process literature." *Clinical Psychology: Science and Practice* 7 (2): 167–88.

2. van Asselt, A. D., C. D. Dirksen, A. Arntz, J. H. Giesen-Bloo, R. van Dyck, P. Spinhoven, W. van Tilburg, I. P. Kremers, M. Nadort, and J. L. Severens. 2008. "Out-patient psychotherapy for borderline personality disorder: Cost-effectiveness of schema-focused therapy v. transference-focused psychotherapy." *British Journal of Psychiatry: The Journal of Mental Science* 192 (6) (June): 450–57.

3. Zanarini, M. C. 2009. "Psychotherapy of borderline personality disorder." *Acta Psychiatrica Scandinavica* 120 (5): 373–77.

CHAPTER 13. THEMES AND VARIATIONS

1. Grant, B. F., F. S. Stinson, D. A. Dawson, S. P. Chou, W. J. Ruan, and R. P. Pickering. 2004. "Co-occurrence of 12-month alcohol and drug use disorders and personality disorders in the United States: Results from the national epidemiologic survey on alcohol and related conditions." *Archives of General Psychiatry* 61 (4) (April 1): 361–68.

2. Goodman, M., U. Patil, L. Steffel, J. Avedon, S. Sasso, J. Triebwasser, and B. Stanley. 2010. "Treatment utilization by gender in patients with borderline personality disorder." *Journal of Psychiatric Practice* 16 (3) (May): 155–63.

3. Johnson, D. M., M. T. Shea, S. Yen, C. L. Battle, C. Zlotnick, C. A. Sanislow, C. M. Grilo, et al. 2003. "Gender differences in borderline personality disorder: Findings from the collaborative longitudinal personality disorders study." *Comprehensive Psychiatry* 44 (4) (July–Aug.): 284–92.

4. McCormick, B., N. Blum, R. Hansel, J. A. Franklin, D. St. John, B. Pfohl, J. Allen, and D. W. Black. 2007. "Relationship of sex to symptom severity, psychiatric comorbidity, and health care utilization in 163 subjects with borderline personality disorder." *Comprehensive Psychiatry* 48 (5) (Sept.–Oct.): 406–12.

5. Tadic, A., S. Wagner, J. Hoch, O. Baskaya, R. von Cube, C. Skaletz, K. Lieb, and N. Dahmen. 2009. "Gender differences in axis I and axis II comorbidity in patients with borderline personality disorder." *Psychopathology* 42 (4): 257–63.

6. American Psychiatric Association. Task Force on DSM-IV. 2000. *Diagnostic and Statistical Manual of Mental Disorders: DSM-IV-TR.* 4th text revision ed. Washington, DC: American Psychiatric Association.

7. Miller, A. L., J. H. Rathus, and M. Linehan. 2007. *Dialectical Behavior Therapy with Suicidal Adolescents.* New York: Guilford Press.

8. Paris, J. 1998. "Personality disorders in sociocultural perspective." *Journal of Personality Disorders* 12 (4) (Winter): 289–301.

9. Castaneda, R., and H. Franco. 1985. "Sex and ethnic distribution of borderline personality disorder in an inpatient sample." *American Journal of Psychiatry* 142 (10): 1202–3.

10. Chavira, D. A., C. M. Grilo, M. T. Shea, S. Yen, J. G. Gunderson, L. C. Morey, A. E. Skodol, R. L. Stout, M. C. Zanarini, and T. H. McGlashan. 2003. "Ethnicity and four personality disorders." *Comprehensive Psychiatry* 44 (6) (Nov.–Dec.): 483–91.

11. Rogler, L. H. 1996. "Framing research on culture in psychiatric diagnosis: The case of the DSM-IV." *Psychiatry* 59 (2) (Summer): 145–55.

12. Kroll, J., K. Carey, L. Sines, and M. Roth. 1982. "Are there borderlines in Britain? A cross-validation of U.S. findings." *Archives of General Psychiatry* 39 (1) (Jan.): 60–63.

13. Moriya, N., Y. Miyake, K. Minakawa, N. Ikuta, and A. Nishizono-Maher. 1993. "Diagnosis and clinical features of borderline personality disorder in the East and West: A preliminary report." *Comprehensive Psychiatry* 34 (6) (Nov.–Dec.): 418–23.

14. Zhong, J., and F. Leung. 2007. "Should borderline personality disorder be included in the fourth edition of the Chinese Classification of Mental Disorders?" *Chinese Medical Journal* 120 (1) (Jan. 5): 77–82.

15. Zhong, J., and F. Leung. 2009. "Diagnosis of borderline personality disorder in China: Current status and future directions." *Current Psychiatry Reports* 11 (1) (Feb.): 69–73.

CHAPTER 14. IF YOU'VE BEEN DIAGNOSED WITH BORDERLINE
PERSONALITY DISORDER

1. Zanarini, M. C., F. R. Frankenburg, D. B. Reich, and G. Fitzmaurice. 2010. "Time to attainment of recovery from borderline personality disorder and stability of recovery: A 10-year prospective follow-up study." *American Journal of Psychiatry* 167 (6) (Apr 15): 618–19.
2. Zanarini, M. C., F. R. Frankenburg, J. Hennen, D. B. Reich, and K. R. Silk. 2004. "Axis I comorbidity in patients with borderline personality disorder: 6-year follow-up and prediction of time to remission." *American Journal of Psychiatry* 161 (11) (Nov.): 2108–14.
3. National Collaborating Centre for Mental Health. 2009. *Borderline Personality Disorder: Treatment and Management.* London: British Psychological Society and the Royal College of Psychiatrists, 68.

CHAPTER 15. FOR PARENTS, PARTNERS, FRIENDS,
AND CO-WORKERS

1. Elliott, B., and O. Weissenborn. 2010. "Employment for persons with borderline personality disorder." *Psychiatric Services* 61 (4) (April 1): 417.
2. Gruys, M. L., and P. R. Sackett. 2003. "Investigating the dimensionality of counterproductive work behavior." *International Journal of Selection and Assessment* 11 (1): 30–42.

APPENDIX B. THEORY AND DEVELOPMENT OF THE
BORDERLINE CONCEPT

1. Kraepelin, E. 1976. *Manic-Depressive Insanity and Paranoia.* Translated by R. Mary Barclay from the 8th German edition of *Textbook of Psychiatry*, vols. 3 and 4, 1920. New York: Arno Press, 130–31.
2. Millon, T., S. Grossman, and S. E. Meagher. 2004. *Masters of the Mind: Exploring the Story of Mental Illness from Ancient Times to the New Millennium.* Hoboken, N.J.: Wiley.
3. Stern, A. 1938. "Psychoanalytic investigation of and therapy in the borderline group of neuroses." *Psychoanalytic Quarterly* 7:467–89.
4. Stone, M. H. 2000. "Clinical guidelines for psychotherapy for patients with borderline personality disorder." *Psychiatric Clinics of North America* 23 (1) (March): 193, 210, ix (including citations).

5. Kernberg, O. F., and R. Michels. 2009. "Borderline personality disorder." *American Journal of Psychiatry* 166 (5) (May 1): 505–8.

6. Masterson, J. F. 1985. *Treatment of the Borderline Adolescent: A Developmental Approach.* New York: Brunner/Mazel.

7. Grinker R. R., B. Werble, R. Drye. 1968. *The Borderline Syndrome: A Behavioral Study of Ego Functions.* New York: Basic Books, 90–91.

8. Gunderson, J. G., and M. T. Singer. 1975. "Defining borderline patients: An overview." *American Journal of Psychiatry* 132 (1) (Jan. 1): 1–10.

9. Gunderson, J. G., and J. E. Kolb. 1978. "Discriminating features of borderline patients." *American Journal of Psychiatry* 135 (7) (July 1): 792–96.

10. Siever, L. J., and K. L. Davis. 1991. "A psychobiological perspective on the personality disorders." *American Journal of Psychiatry* 148 (12) (Dec. 1): 1647–58.

11. Skodol, A. E., J. G. Gunderson, M. T. Shea, T. H. McGlashan, L. C. Morey, C. A. Sanislow, D. S. Bender, et al. 2005. "The Collaborative Longitudinal Personality Disorders Study (CLPS): Overview and implications." *Journal of Personality Disorders* 19 (5) (Oct.): 487–504.

12. Zanarini, M. C., F. R. Frankenburg, J. Hennen, D. B. Reich, and K. R. Silk. 2005. "The McLean Study of Adult Development (MSAD): Overview and implications of the first six years of prospective follow-up." *Journal of Personality Disorders* 19 (5) (Oct.): 505–23.

13. Gunderson, J. G. 2009. "Borderline personality disorder: Ontogeny of a diagnosis." *American Journal of Psychiatry* 166 (5) (May 1): 530–39.

INDEX

"Abandonment depression," 263
Abandonment fears, 10, 17, 263
Abilify (aripiprazole), 149
Abuse history. *See* Trauma history
Abusive behaviors, 239–43. *See also* Aggression
Action stage of change, 157
Adderall, 93
Addictions. *See* Substance abuse
Adolescents with borderline personality traits, 196–205, 263; dialectical behavior therapy for, 200–205; distress of, 199; family involvement in treatment of, 199–200, 201–3, 240; identification of, 197–98; psychoeducation about, 201–2; social role of, 198, 200; symptom persistence in, 198–99; symptom severity in, 198; validating behaviors and feelings of, 203–5
Aggression, 152, 154, 195, 237–38, 239. *See also* Abusive behaviors
Agreeableness, 75, 77; in BPD, 78, 79
Alcoholics Anonymous, 226
Alcoholism, 5–6, 18, 32, 44–45, 88–91, 113; accurate reporting of, 225; self-harm and, 238
Alcohol withdrawal, 151, 225–26
Allport, Gordon, 73
Alprazolam (Xanax), 151–52
Altruline (sertraline), 139
American Psychiatric Association (APA), 135, 137
Amitriptyline (Elavil), 141
Amoxapine (Asendin), 141
Amphetamine abuse, 92–93
Amygdala, 65–68, 71
Anafranil (clomipramine), 141

Anger/rage, 10, 59, 79, 82, 138, 260, 264; abusive behavior and, 239–43; in adolescents, 198; lamotrigine for, 63–64, 148; in workplace, 246
Anhedonia, 30, 52
Anorexia nervosa, 32, 46, 97, 98–100; understanding, 101–3
Antianxiety medications, 150–52
Antidepressants, xiii, 29, 51, 79, 137, 138–45; effectiveness of, 138; monoamine oxidase inhibitors, 142–44; selective serotonin reuptake inhibitors, 138–40; tetracyclic, 140; tricyclic, 140–42
Antipsychotics: atypical, 137, 148–50; phenothiazines, 148
Antisocial behaviors, 195–96
Antisocial personality disorder, 241
Anxiety, 13, 14, 15, 59, 79, 82, 261; benzodiazepines for, 94, 150–52; psychotherapy-precipitated, 178
APA (American Psychiatric Association), 135, 137
Appetite changes, 52, 56
Aremis (sertraline), 139
Arguments, 241
Aripiprazole (Abilify), 149
Aropax (Paroxetine), 139
Asenapine (Saphris), 149
Asendin (amoxapine), 141
Association studies, 71
Ataque de nervios, 206–7
Automatic thoughts, 164
Axelrod, Julius, 138

Beck, Aaron, 160–63
Behavior(s): abusive, 239–43; consequences of, 240, 241–42; definition of, 87; reckless,